ROBERT W. SEARS, M.D., AND **JAMES M. SEARS, M.D.**
THE CO-AUTHORS OF *THE BABY BOOK*

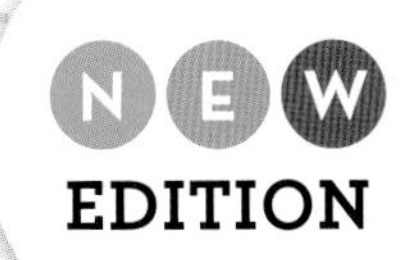

25 Things Every New Dad Should Know

Essential First Steps for Fathers

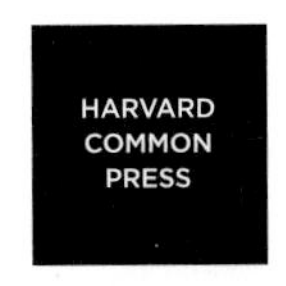

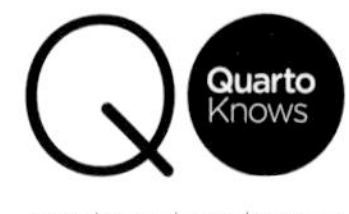

First Published in 2017 by The Harvard Common Press, an imprint of The Quarto Group,
100 Cummings Center, Suite 265-D, Beverly, MA 01915, USA.
T (978) 282-9590 F (978) 283-2742 QuartoKnows.com

The Harvard Common Press titles are also available at discount for retail, wholesale, promotional, and bulk purchase. For details, contact the Special Sales Manager by email at specialsales@quarto.com or by mail at The Quarto Group, Attn: Special Sales Manager, 401 Second Avenue North, Suite 310, Minneapolis, MN 55401, USA.

21 20 19 18 17 1 2 3 4 5

ISBN: 978-1-55832-893-8

Digital edition published in 2017

Originally found under the following Library of Congress Cataloging-in-Publication Data

Sears, Robert, M.D.
Father's first steps : 25 things every new dad should know / Robert W. Sears and
James M. Sears ; foreword by William Sears.
p. cm.
ISBN 1-55832-335-X (hardcover : alk. paper)
1. Fathers—Life skills guides. 2. Fatherhood. 3. Infants—Care. 4. Father and infant.
I. Sears, James M. II. Title.
HQ756.S397 2006
306.874'2—dc22 2005035169
ISBN-13: 978-1-55832-335-3
ISBN-10: 1-55832-335-X

Printed in China

For our children who taught us everything we know.

For our wives who remind us of everything we forget.

And for our parents who made us who we are today.

Contents

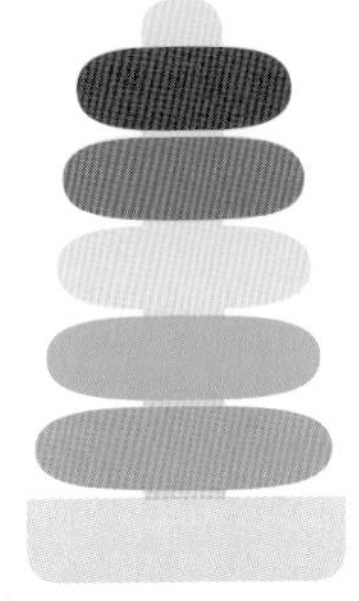

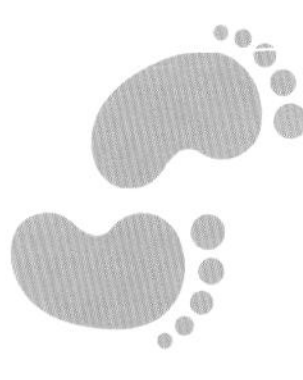

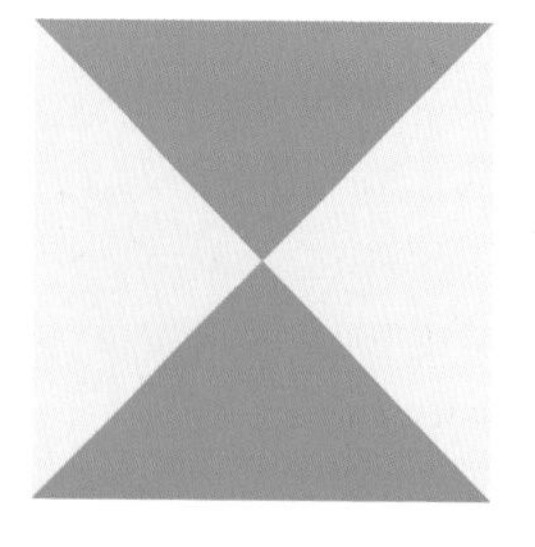

Foreword

It's a dad's dream to write the introduction to a book written by his sons!

One day I was scheduled to give an evening talk to a group of expectant dads. Earlier that day an expectant mom in our office asked me, "How do I get my husband to attend your talk? This is our first baby, and I want him to get prepared." I suggested she tell him that they were going to attend a talk about some new and exciting investments they could make. The expectant dad responded with my two favorite words for a happy marriage, "Yes, dear!" and off to the talk they went. The couple sat in the front row, and within a few minutes I saw him nudge his wife and say, "I thought he was going to talk about investments. He's talking about babies!" At the end of the talk, the father thanked me. He had just realized that he was about to make the best investment of his life.

Imagine that you're about to start a new job. You're naturally apprehensive because you may have had no training for this job. It requires new skills and new tools. Consider this book to be like your first toolbox, a set of beginner tools that will help you put more into your investment, so that years down the road you'll be able to sit back and enjoy your returns. In this new job you may have to start at the bottom—learning how to change diapers. You will be frustrated at times that your wife seems to know instinctively what to do. You will learn how to handle a crying baby when your wife says, "Here, I've had it! You try to calm him!" Comforting fussy babies is where dads can really shine, and Dr. Bob and Dr. Jim will show you how. Instead of fumbling around, you will comfort your baby and score lots of points with your wife. Nothing turns on a woman like seeing a big man nurture a tiny baby.

Throughout this book, Dr. Bob and Dr. Jim give you tools to help your baby trust you as a nurturer. You are not just a pinch hitter, filling in for Mom. Your children will enjoy the different ways you parent them, the way you talk, the way you hold them, and the way you play with them. It's not greater or less than what Mom does. It's different, and children thrive on this difference. Dr. Bob and Dr. Jim want you to be the best dad you can be, and they will show you how. Using their combined almost 50 years of fathering, they share with you what they've learned works for most dads most of the time.

Raising eight children has helped me mature into a better man, a better husband, and a better person, and I have watched my sons grow with their own families. Even though I taught Bob and Jim everything they know (or so I like to think), their experiences with their own five kids have allowed them to build and expand on this knowledge to share unique insights with you. Throughout this book the authors bleed a bit. They've made mistakes and learned from them, and they've learned from their wives. The 25 tips they offer you throughout this book are sure to help you enjoy the fulfilling rewards of investing your time and person into your baby.

As I've seen each of my children grow up, move out, get married, start their careers, and have children, it's been a true joy to look back to the very beginning and remember the countless hours I spent holding, walking, rocking, changing, dressing, and playing with each one of my babies. As I look at my relationship with my older kids, I know my investment has paid off a hundredfold. Dr. Bob and Dr. Jim will help your life investment pay off for you and your kids as well.

—Dr. Bill Sears

A First Word to Dad

You're about to become a father. Or maybe you have your new bundle of joy already. Maybe you're holding this book because your wife, girlfriend, mother-in-law, or a well-intentioned friend thinks you need it. If so, don't take it personally. Somebody was probably just looking for a cute present and thought you'd be more likely to read a short book than a whole encyclopedia on parenting. Anyway, your wife will read all the important books and fill you in on what you need to know, right?

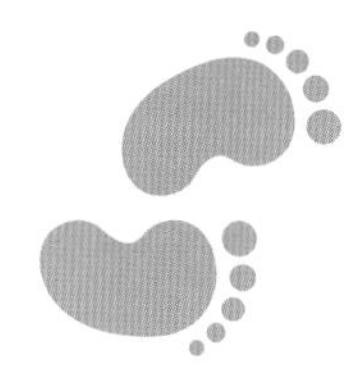

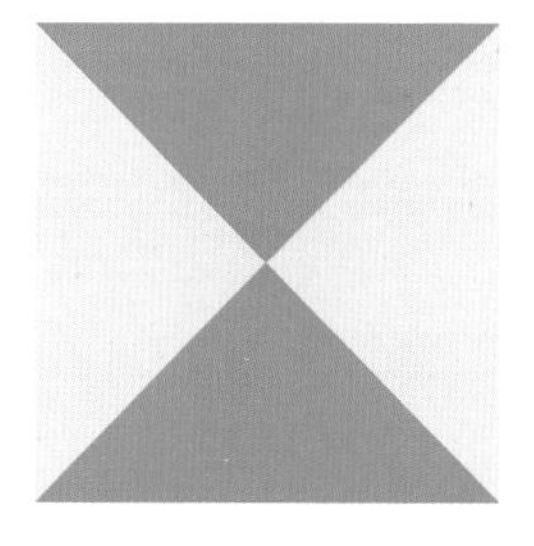

Maybe. But as a new dad you don't want to risk being left out of the loop, do you? You want to be just as prepared as your baby's mother, but you want the short version, the Spark Notes, the facts you need to know without all the extra stuff. That's what *25 Things Every New Dad Should Know* is all about.

Now, are there really only 25 things you need to know as you start your new role as a dad? Of course not. We've sneaked a lot more than that into this book. But being a father is a learn-as-you-go job anyway. There's no book in the world that can completely prepare you for what you are about to experience—not because there is so much information involved, but because you and your baby are unique. No author, not even these two, can anticipate everything your new baby is going to bring out in you as a dad. Fathering isn't a test you can study for. Let your baby teach you what you need to know along the way. We're just here to offer a few tips, tell a few jokes, and share what we've learned along our own journeys through fatherhood.

So relax, grab a drink and some chips and salsa, sit out on the lawn chair in your backyard, and spend an afternoon absorbing what we feel are the most useful ideas and insights that will help you start on the right path as a new father.

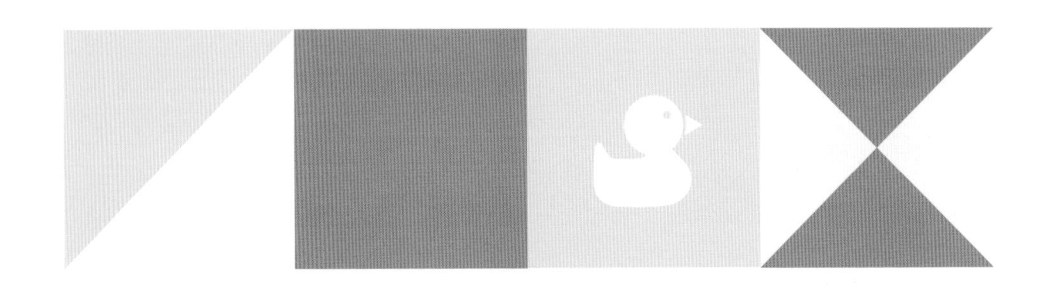

A Note to Women

So you're thinking about buying this book for your husband, son, son-in-law, friend, or boyfriend? There's a man in your life who's about to take the big plunge into fatherhood, and you are looking for a way to ease him into his new responsibilities.

You've come to the right place. *25 Things Every New Dad Should Know* is the ultimate guide to becoming a new father. We can't tell the dad-to-be how to be a great dad; he'll need to discover that within himself. But we'll help him find his own fatherliness, develop his own parenting instincts, and unleash the hidden dad within. We'll challenge him to be the best father and mate he can be.

Exactly what kind of advice are we going to give him? Well, you could read the book before he does to make sure you agree with what we're going to tell him. Or you could just trust us, and trust *him*, and then sit back and watch what happens when he gets his hands on that new baby.

Don't worry. This book has been "approved" by our wives, our own mom, and several other experienced moms. You can feel confident that this new dad will be getting some good advice.

You may be worried for nothing. He may surprise you. Having a baby suddenly thrust into his arms may bring about an immediate transformation. Nothing turns a tough guy into a blob of mush better than a little squirming baby. You don't have to make a man be a good dad; a baby brings it out in him. We're here just to give him a little nudge if needed.

We'll be thankful for the privilege of sharing our thoughts with the new dad in your life.

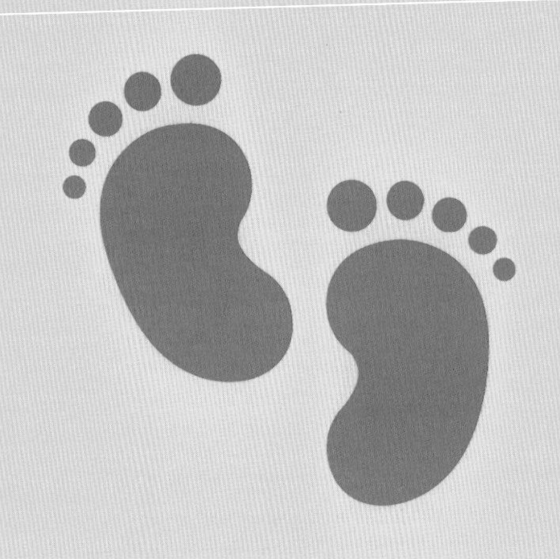

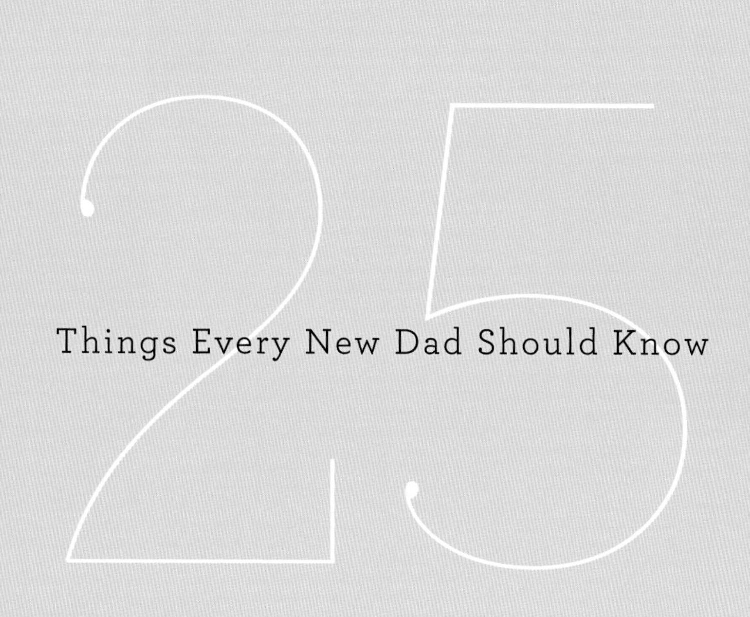

25 Things Every New Dad Should Know

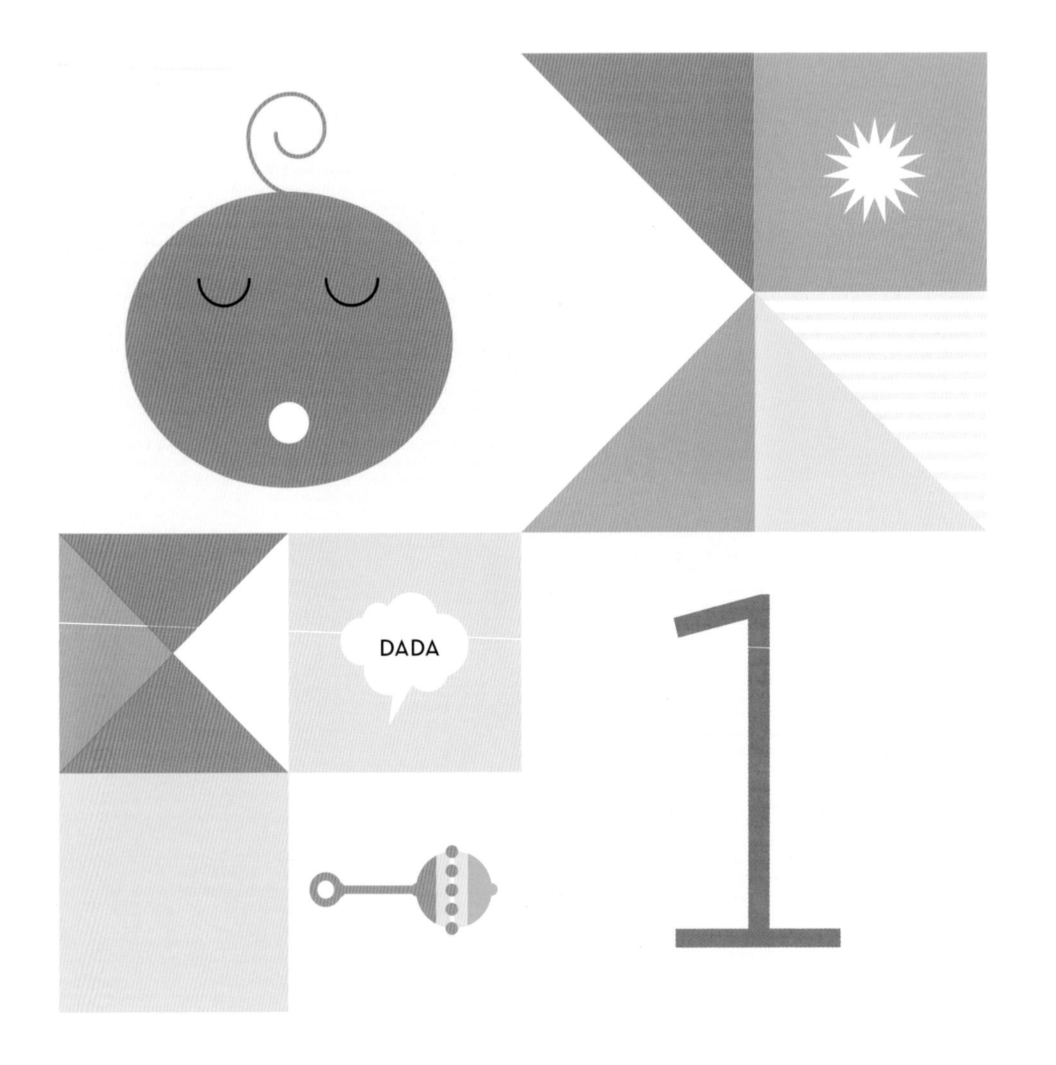
DADA
1

Real Dads Change Diapers

Your baby was born just a few hours ago. You and the new mom have been through a lot over the past nine months (well, *she* has, anyway—your main involvement lasted for about 15 minutes). Mom is sleeping. Your new baby lies in the bassinet. He or she looks around at the new world. You beam with pride as you watch your new bundle of joy. You dream about teaching the little one to throw a ball, ride a bike, do a somersault, play video games, drive a car. This baby is your offspring. He or she will carry your name forward. And eventually the grandchildren will carry it, too. This child is your immortality. Life is good. You notice a funny grin on the baby's face. . . .

Whoa, what is that smell? He has a diaperful.

Looking around, you hope someone else will take care of it. Where is that nurse when you need her? You glance at Mom, but she is sleeping for the first time in 39 hours. You won't start teaching your child how to throw a baseball for another two years, and you figured Mom would take care of all the baby stuff until then. Should you wake her up? Go right ahead, and she'll probably never forgive you. What you do with this diaper could define you as a dad. Will you jump in, get your hands dirty, and become an attached, involved father? Or will you just sit back through the baby years and wait until your son's throwing arm is in shape?

Reading this, you are probably thinking, "Hold on, it's only one stinking diaper!" You're right. It is only a diaper. And, yes, it stinks. But if you really think about it—deeply think about it, in a Zen sort of way—this is much more than a diaper change. This is your chance to take fatherhood by the horns and run with it! Now is your chance to rise above the media's perception that all dads are inept, football-watching, beer-drinking Homer Simpsons who are completely clueless when it comes to taking care of a baby.

Exactly how do you change a diaper anyway? We're not going to tell you, not yet. Despite its title, this chapter isn't about *how* to change a diaper. It's about *wanting* to change a diaper, or at least deciding to change a diaper even when you don't want to. In chapter 8 we'll give you step-by-step instructions so you can change a diaper like a pro. But who cares that you're an amateur right now?

At least your wife will see you make the attempt. Even if she sleeps through your efforts, the nurse may come in and take notice, and later on tell Mom that you did your duty dutifully. And if nobody sees you trying to be a good dad, that's OK, too. You'll have your first little father-baby bonding experience, and you'll be able to say to yourself, "Hey, I can do this whole dad thing."

Changing the first diaper doesn't really take any skill anyway; it takes only a desire to make a difference in this little one's life. To be there for him. To be willing to get your hands a little messy. To take a little time on this first day, and every single day for the next 18 years, to give your child some hands-on attention.

Your child will have many needs and tasks throughout life that he can't accomplish alone. You can start right now in giving him the message "I am here for you—no matter what." This is a message he will learn to count on for the rest of his life. "I am here for you when you need your diaper changed. I am here for you when you trip and bump your head. I am here for you when you fall off the jungle gym. I am here with you when the other kids in class tease you about your new haircut. When I get home from work, exhausted, and you ask me to take you on a bike ride, we will ride like the wind. I will be here for you when you get into trouble at school. I will support you as much as I can when you try out for the team. I will be cheering loudest even when you lose the state championship. I will risk my life when I first let you take the wheel of the family car. I will do what I can when your entire world comes crashing down because your first love wants to be just friends."

Be a hands-on father. This will be the best investment of your life.

Sorry, we're getting a little ahead of ourselves. Forget about the teenage years for now; let's just focus on today. Studies show that 75 percent of dads will pretend not to notice a dirty diaper to avoid having to change it. If you read this figure in a magazine you'd probably think to yourself, "I can't believe so many dads sink that low. I'll never be that way." Now's your chance to prove it.

Diaper changing is hands-on fathering. The more times you touch your kids, whether through diaper changes, hugs, or games of catch, the better you will know them. Your child will need 5,000 diaper changes over the next few years. This adds up to about 250 hours of one-on-one time getting to know your child.

Many dads shy away not only from changing diapers but from all the mundane duties of baby care. You may figure Mom is better at swaddling, cuddling, and consoling, and so you let her do it all. But the more you let mom do *everything*, the less involved you become as a father. Eventually you will have some major catch-up to do. Dads, we urge you to change that diaper. Be a hands-on father. This will be the best investment of your life. The rest of this book will give you many tools (Tools? Cool!) you can use to be the world's greatest dad. Start with that first diaper, and you'll be well on your way.

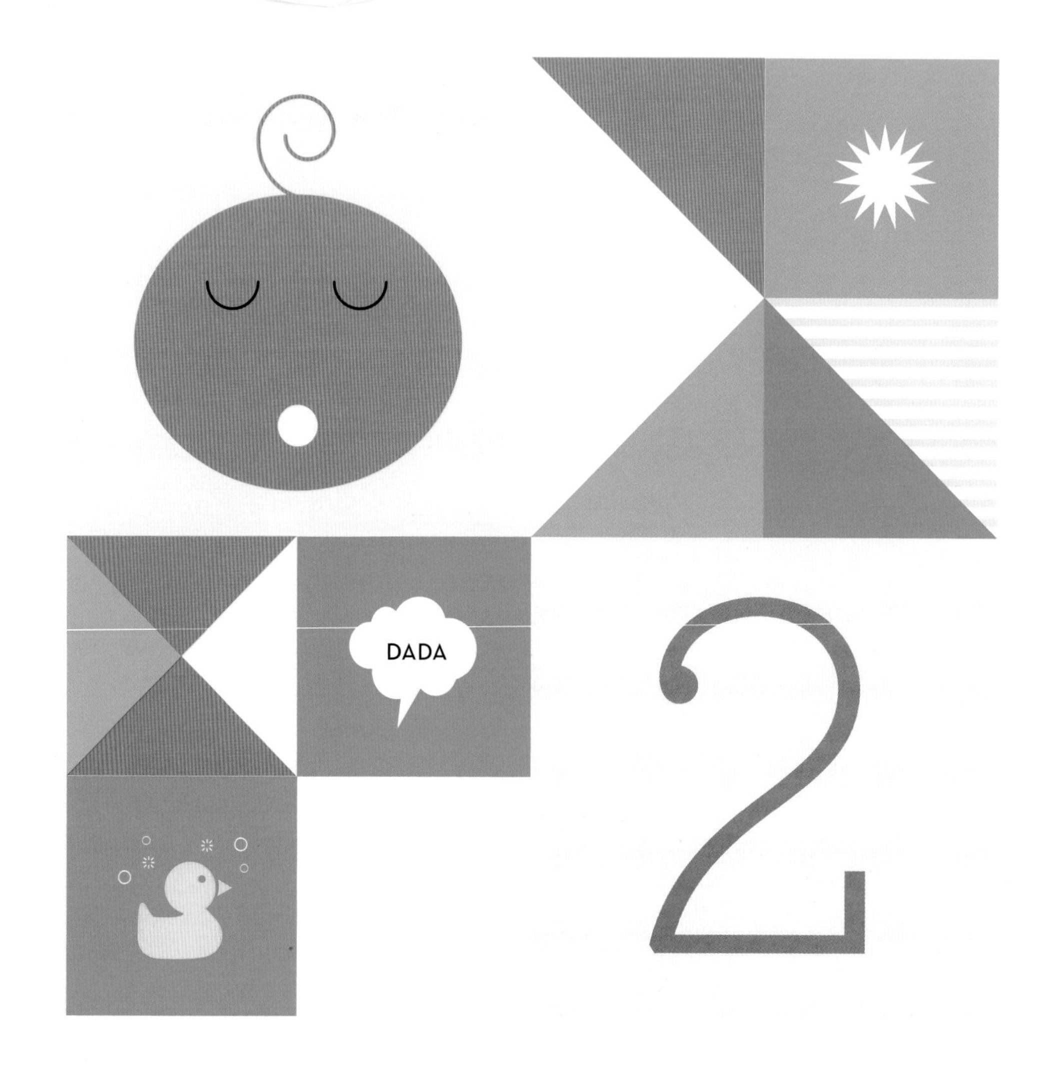
DADA

You're a Key Player on the Birth Team

It's almost here: the Big Day you and your mate have spent nine months waiting for. As you anticipate the birth of your baby, here is your heads-up on what you can expect and how best to prepare for the event. Take it from two dads who have been there five times with their own wives and countless times with other new parents: Having a baby will probably be the biggest life-changing event of your life. If you have already gone through the birth process with your spouse, don't skip this chapter. You may find our ideas interesting, and we promise a joke or two to make it worth your while.

Remember how on your wedding day everyone joked that it was *her* day? That it was all about *her*, and that you were there just to tag along? Well, don't let anyone tell you the same thing about the birth of your baby. You can experience the joy of birth as much as any new mom can. Set other cares aside, and focus all your attention on your wife while she labors and births your baby.

Helping a woman through labor is much more than coaching her through breathing and pushing. She needs to feel you are connected to her 100 percent, both emotionally and physically. Physical support means standing by her side, placing your hands on her, sitting behind her for support, and feeding her ice chips and sips of juice. It means ignoring distractions like the TV. Most labor-and-delivery rooms have a television, and we've always wondered why. Is it so Dad can watch the ball game while the nurses help Mom through labor? We've actually caught some dads doing just that! Turn it off! Have a buddy record the game so you can watch it next week. Emotional support means listening to everything the new mom says, answering and even anticipating her needs, flooding her with words of encouragement and support, and clearing your mind of concerns about work or finances.

You may think you will be too overwhelmed to be that pillar of support your mate needs on this special day. One way you can free yourself to enjoy the birth experience is to hire professional help. You're probably thinking, "We already have! We have the best O.B. in the city, and we've chosen the best hospital in the county. We have all the professional help we need." We're talking about a professional labor support person, or doula. If you and your mate are planning a home birth or using a birthing center, you already have a midwife who will provide support through labor, and perhaps you have a doula as well. In the hospital, though, the O.B. is there only to make sure there are no medical complications and to guide the baby out of the birth canal, a process that usually takes about 20 minutes. The O.B. doesn't support the mom through the hours or days of labor. A labor-and-delivery nurse will guide her through the really active part of labor and pushing, and this nurse will be well trained and helpful. If the labor-and-delivery unit is unexpectedly busy, though, the nurse may not be able to give your wife the close attention she needs. Besides, your wife has no personal connection with this nurse—they have probably never even met before. This leaves you.

Now, if you are one of those supermen who actually pays attention in prenatal classes, knows everything about labor, and is ready to coach a woman through position changes, breathing patterns, and relaxation techniques to give her the birthing experience she wants, then we applaud you. But if you belong to the other 99 percent of men, you probably have no idea what to expect, much less how to guide your partner through it. That's how Dr. Bob felt with his first baby:

"We hired a doula several months before the due date. She formed a relationship with my wife so she would know exactly what Cheryl needed during labor. I left the doula in charge of knowing when to have Cheryl walk around and when to suggest she lie down, how to guide her breathing (is it 'hee hee hoo' or

'hoo hoo hee'?), and what positions to get in to make the contractions easier. This freed me up to just experience the birth process with my wife and to be there for her—giving back rubs, helping her walk and change positions, wiping her sweaty brow, keeping her hydrated, and doing anything else she wanted or needed."

Immerse yourself in the emotional experience of childbirth, and you'll be better prepared to receive that tiny little baby into your world.

Dr. Jim and his wife were also glad they hired a doula:

"During our childbirth classes, I tried to learn as much as I could about being the 'Dad-coach.' But then a thought occurred to me: Wouldn't it be better to have a coach who has done this before? Giving birth would be my wife's crowning achievement—her Super Bowl—and I don't think that any team would try to go to the big game with a leader who has never coached before. So we hired a professional. Our doula had coached hundreds of times. She knew the people on the hospital staff—their strengths and weaknesses—and she helped us get one of the better nurses. This freed me to play the role I was more suited for: Nervous New Dad. In addition to wiping my wife's brow and holding her hand, I fetched fresh ice chips and warm blankets (the doula told me where the nurses were hiding them)."

If you can't hire a labor assistant, bring along your wife's closest friend or family member to lend emotional support, and let the professionals at the hospital guide you through. If your prenatal classes haven't started yet, be sure to attend, and to pay attention. We know some dads who have been outstanding labor coaches, and you can be one, too.

"But who's going to record the birth?" you may ask. Definitely not you! It's hard for most guys to give up this all-important job, but trust us: You need to have a friend or a family member act as cinematographer for the day. If you want to keep your phone or a small camera in your pocket for the occasional snapshot, go ahead. But don't let the camera get in the way. Besides, don't you want to be in all the pictures so you can show your kids in later years what a supportive and excited new dad you were?

If you focus completely on the process of labor and birth, you will feel as if you're experiencing it yourself (well, almost—you won't get to enjoy as much physical work or actual pain). You will be emotionally prepared to receive your new baby with open arms. A new mom is usually flooded with emotion when her new baby is placed on her belly, but we often see Dad just stand there and watch. Get your hands on your new baby. Snuggle up to Mom, and let the tears flow.

Your life is about to change. Get ready to change with it! Don't be a stand-back dad; be a stand-up man on this special day. Immerse yourself in the emotional experience of childbirth, and you'll be better prepared to receive that tiny little baby into your world. What do you do if you really aren't feeling an immediate emotional attachment to your new baby? Maybe you just aren't one of those touchy-feely kind of men who cried at the end of *Casablanca*. Sure, you're excited, but you just aren't *feeling* it. If the labor and delivery process didn't suck you in, don't worry. We have the cure, and it's just about to be placed in your arms. Turn the page, and get ready to be a dad.

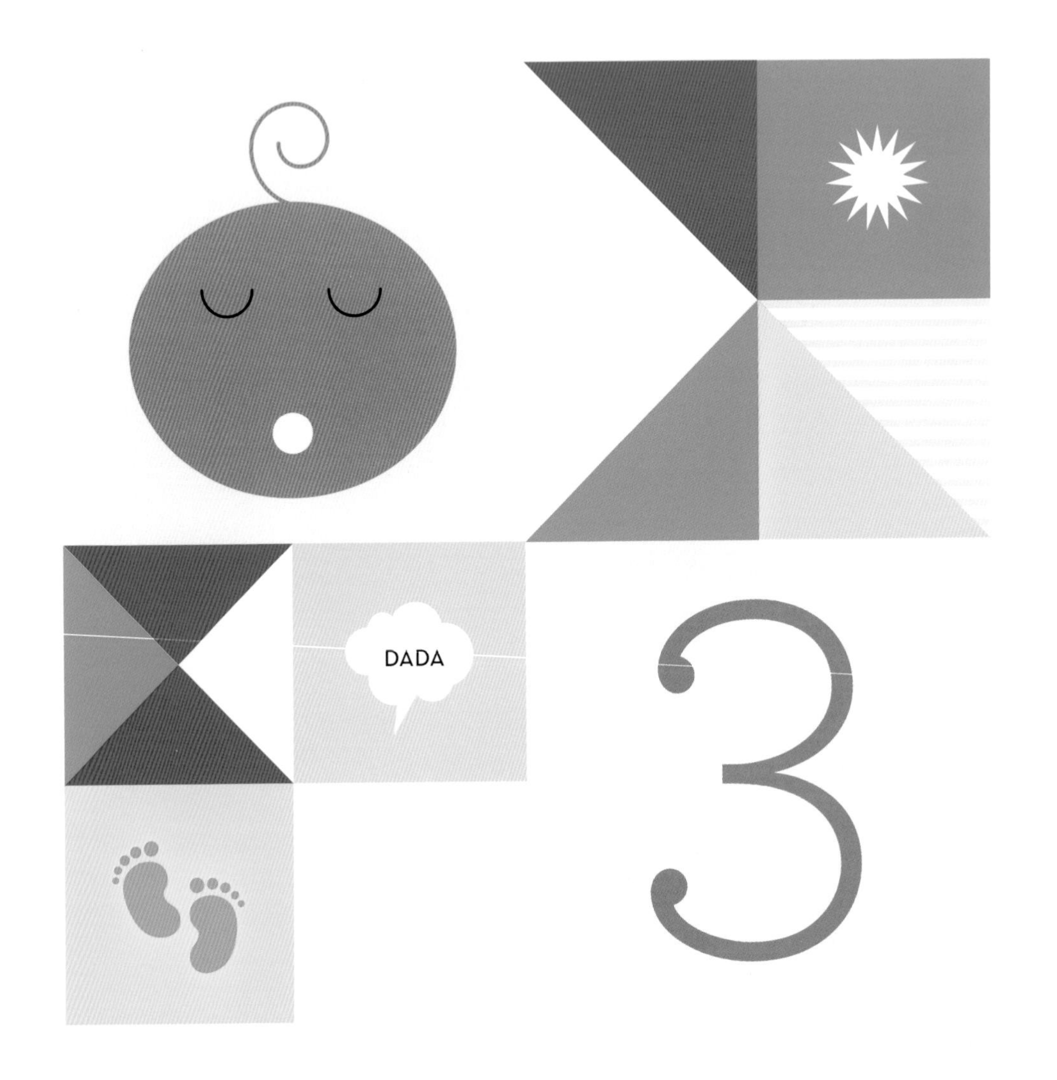
DADA
3

You and Your Baby Will Need Some Super Glue

Now that you have a new baby, you are probably wondering, "What kind of dad will I be?" We're going to assume that you want to be a good dad, or maybe even a great dad. If you are reading this book because your wife or mother-in-law insists, and you were really just hoping to be a mediocre dad, then this chapter isn't for you. But most people are always searching for the secret to success. They're looking for that quick and easy road to becoming the best in their field. Now that you're a new dad, how can you become the best dad there ever was? Or at least make the Top 10?

There is only one thing you have to do to ensure that every other aspect of fatherhood falls neatly into place. There's a secret handshake, so to speak; if you master it, you will be welcomed into the Best Dads in the World Club. This thing is very simple, yet intricately complex. It's easy to do, yet it will occupy a lot of your time. You don't need to study up or read any directions (who wants to read directions, anyway?). There's no remote control involved, and no assembly is required. What exactly is this secret?

All you have to do is hold your baby.

"That's it?" you ask. "That's the big secret? It sounds too easy. There's gotta be more. Give me a list with at least three main bullet points, or five steps to follow. Any good plan has at least five steps."

Actually, no. Being a great dad comes down to one basic concept—bonding. Approach fatherhood in the same way you approach problems around the house, whether you're fixing something that's broken or building something from scratch. Use Super Glue. Duct tape also works. You've got to stick yourself to your baby.

No, wait, come back and sit down. Don't actually get the glue. We're using a metaphor. Let us explain clearly.

The more you hold your baby, the better your baby will get to know you. She'll learn your touch, your smell, your voice, and your breath. She'll become so familiar with you that she'll crave your contact.

But how does this make you a better dad? The baby isn't the only one who benefits from bonding. Holding your baby will help bring out the best in you as well. We'll tell you in chapter 22 about the hormonal changes that bring out the new mom's mothering instincts. A new dad also undergoes hormonal changes that urge him to respond to his baby. Every time you give in to this urge, you learn more about your baby—how she breathes, how she moves, what each type of cry means. The more time you spend consoling your baby during fussy periods, interacting face-to-face with her during playful times, and holding her while she naps, the better you get to know her, and the more trust she develops in you to meet her needs. You also learn to trust yourself, and this builds your confidence as a dad. You will carry this confidence throughout your many decades as a parent. Later, this confidence will help you make all (or mostly all) the right parenting decisions.

In the course of writing this book, Dr. Bob made an interesting observation:

"I walked into an exam room to do a one-week checkup on a little baby. Dad was standing there holding the baby while the little one sucked on Dad's finger. While I examined the baby, Dad stood nearby with his hand on the baby's head. The baby pooped, and the dad changed the diaper. Then the baby got hungry, and the dad, without any prompting from Mom, ran to get the nursing pillow from the car. He placed the pillow on Mom's lap, then handed over the baby. What was Mom doing the whole time? Sitting there talking to me about how she was adjusting to the new baby. With all this fatherly support, I knew that this mom and baby were in good hands."

Here's what Dr. Bob did after his first baby was born:

"I did almost nothing but hold him. When my wife wasn't feeding him, when Grandma and Grandpa weren't holding him, I held him. I spent every waking hour I could holding him. Why did I do this? Because I was jealous. I was jealous of the incredible bond my wife was building with our baby through breastfeeding. She was getting to know him so well, and I knew that I would miss out on something amazing if I didn't jump in and get involved. This was a pivotal moment in my life as a new dad. I could either stand back and let my wife enjoy all the bonding, or I could join the club. Boy, am I ever glad I joined. People talk about a mother's intuition, but I believe that I developed an intuition about each of our children just as deep as my wife's."

If you choose to develop a close bond with your baby, we want to warn you about something. You are going to hear from your parents, in-laws, other family members, or friends that you are spoiling the baby. "Don't hold that baby too much." "You'll never be able to put her down." "She'll never learn to be independent."

Thankfully, such old-fashioned ideas have been proven wrong. Researchers at numerous universities across the United States have found that infants who are held more grow faster, show accelerated intellectual and motor development, and become more happily independent after infancy. In just about any aspect of life, when something is lovingly cared for, it grows and thrives. When it is left alone to fend for itself, it spoils. This is doubly true for babies.

Researchers at numerous universities across the United States have found that infants who are held more grow faster, show accelerated intellectual and motor development, and become more happily independent after infancy. In just about any aspect of life, when something is lovingly cared for, it grows and thrives.

Don't let anyone—including us—tell you to treat your baby in a way that goes against your instincts. You and your baby's mother—not your in-laws and not your friends—are the only ones who can truly judge what is best for you and your baby. You are responsible for the relationship you create. Trust yourself and your instincts. Create a bond with your baby that allows these instincts to develop and thrive.

Tragically, parents who don't form close bonds with their babies, out of fear of spoiling, don't enjoy as close a relationship when their child grows older and more independent. Dr. Bob understood this right away with his first baby:

"My wife was going to 'spoil' our baby whether I helped or not, so I figured I might as well be just as close to our spoiled baby as my wife was going to be."

Dr. Jim cringes when new parents in the office tell him they don't want to hold the baby too much:

"'We don't want her to become too attached to us,' they say. Then I know I am in for a lengthy discussion in which I'll attempt to open their minds to a new way of thinking.

"I usually start at the end of the story. I ask, 'Do you know any parents of teenagers who complain that their teens are too attached to Mom and Dad?' I sure don't. In 15 years, the parents who avoid holding their baby now will be scratching their heads, wondering why they can't communicate with their rebellious, self-centered teenager. The old model of parenting follows these rules: Don't get too tied to your young baby; don't hold her too much; try to get her to be independent as soon as possible . . . and then try to reverse all this when she hits junior high.

"In my experience with patients and my own kids, almost all teenagers go through a normal and healthy time of distancing themselves from their parents, both physically and emotionally. If parents bond well with their newborn and stay close to her throughout childhood, they will enjoy a well-adjusted, self-confident, trustful teenager who is emotionally connected to Mom and Dad—even though she doesn't want to be seen with them at the mall."

You may wonder how you are supposed to get anything done around the house if you're holding the baby all the time. This is where you have to be creative. Get used to "wearing" your baby in a carrier of some sort. When our babies were small, we preferred a sling, because it let us switch among various positions depending on what we were doing. We could have both hands free if we needed to open a can of soup or type on the computer. We've even managed to write books with babies slung on our laps.

Admittedly, your mother-in-law is right about one thing. If you hold your baby a lot, she will want to be held a lot. She'll want as much of a good thing as she can get. But if you are committed to developing a close bond with your baby, and are willing to put in plenty of holding time in the early months, you won't regret it in the long run.

Don't be afraid to glue yourself to your baby. Establish a bond so strong that you and your child will cherish it your entire lives.

DADA
4

Your Baby Needs Your Little Finger

There is a lot that happens in the hospital after birth besides bonding. Maybe you don't want to know about this; a lot of people are uncomfortable when it comes to doctors and hospitals. But you're a man. You can take it. You're not afraid of a needle or two, are you?

Anyway, you're not the patient now. Your *child* is.

A hospital can be a scary place for any newborn. Your baby has just spent the last nine months in a warm, soothing womb. For him, being thrown into the bright lights, stuck with sharp needles, pressed with cold stethoscopes, and prodded with thermometers is unpleasant and sometimes downright painful.

Why does it matter if the baby is poked and prodded until he cries? Well, in the long run, it probably doesn't matter too much. Babies do get over this treatment. But a lot goes on in a baby's first few days. He must learn to nurse. He must begin bonding with his parents. His physiology—temperature, breathing, heart rate, and nervous system—must learn to regulate itself. And his entire transition from life inside the womb to life outside goes better if he is comfortable, content, and calm.

The question you must ask yourself is this: Are you going to let your baby cry his way through the first two days of life while he endures various hospital procedures? Or are you going to try to minimize the intrusions, comfort him through it all, and help make his transition into this world a little more gentle?

It's not easy to ask a medical practitioner, "Is this procedure really necessary? Is there a way to make it more comfortable? Can it wait a little while until the baby is settled down a bit?" As a father, you will be standing up for your child almost every day. You'll be insisting that the soccer coach put your kid in the game, and that your teenage daughter's boyfriend keep his paws off her. Why not stand up for your child on day one?

You will meet hospital personnel who are sympathetic and respectful of your wishes, but you may meet others who try to brush you aside. "Oh, don't worry," they may say. "Babies are tough. They don't mind." Well, then, why is your baby screaming at the top of his lungs while the nurse is drawing his blood? Others may say, "He'll be fine. He won't remember this anyway." That makes your baby feel a whole lot better, doesn't it?

For the rest of your child's life, doctors, nurses, and dentists will be telling him, "Don't worry, this won't hurt a bit." When he is older, your child can choose whether or not to believe this. Right now, you have to be the one to step forward. It's OK to be like Dr. Bob:

"I was one of those parents who questioned everything until the nurses rolled their eyes. If they had to do something to my baby, I was going to comfort him through it."

So, what kind of comfort can you provide? Research has shown that when babies are held skin-to-skin against a parent's chest during any procedure, they feel less pain. So when the nurse comes in to draw the baby's blood, whip off your shirt, hold the baby to your chest, and tell the nurse to go for it. And seriously, research has shown that babies who are nursed before and after a procedure feel even less discomfort. So maybe let Mom do the snuggling.

Of course, it's not always practical for Mom to breastfeed the baby through every painful intrusion, but giving him something else to suck on is almost as good. Here's something Dr. Bob learned with his first baby:

"He loved to suck on my finger. So any time someone wanted to do something to him, I would snuggle up to his head and put my well-washed pinky into his mouth. Between my finger and my wife's breasts, we made the hospital stay much easier for the little guy."

To successfully fill in for the breast, you need to know three secrets to finger suckling: First, most babies like the pinky the best, since it's about the same size as Mom's nipple. Second, you have to turn your palm up so the fingernail is on your baby's tongue instead of the roof of his mouth (make sure that the nail is clean and short). Finally, you need to let the baby suck in your finger all the way to the second knuckle, just as he sucks in more of the breast than just the nipple. If the baby gags, pull back a bit.

We examine many new babies in the hospital every week. Because we have to unwrap and undress them, they often cry during part of the exam. One of our favorite scenes occurs when the new mom is disturbed by the baby's protests but can't easily get up to put a hand on her baby. Mom will glare at Dad and nod her head forcefully in the baby's direction, and finally it will dawn on Dad to go over and offer his baby some comfort. Even better is when Dad does this without any prompting from Mom. When we see that, we know Dad is hooked.

Some new dads and moms are more relaxed about hospitals. They don't seem to mind the intrusions and trust that everything the doctors and nurses are doing for the baby is for the best. No matter how upset the baby may get, they know it won't last long. But we worry about parents who aren't bothered when their babies are in pain. Are they so relaxed that nothing ever fazes them, or are they not yet bonding with the new baby?

If you think you may not be forming that bond just yet, don't worry. It's only day one. Just pour on a little more glue, change a few more diapers, and soon no one will be able to pry your baby out of your arms, much less prick him with a needle.

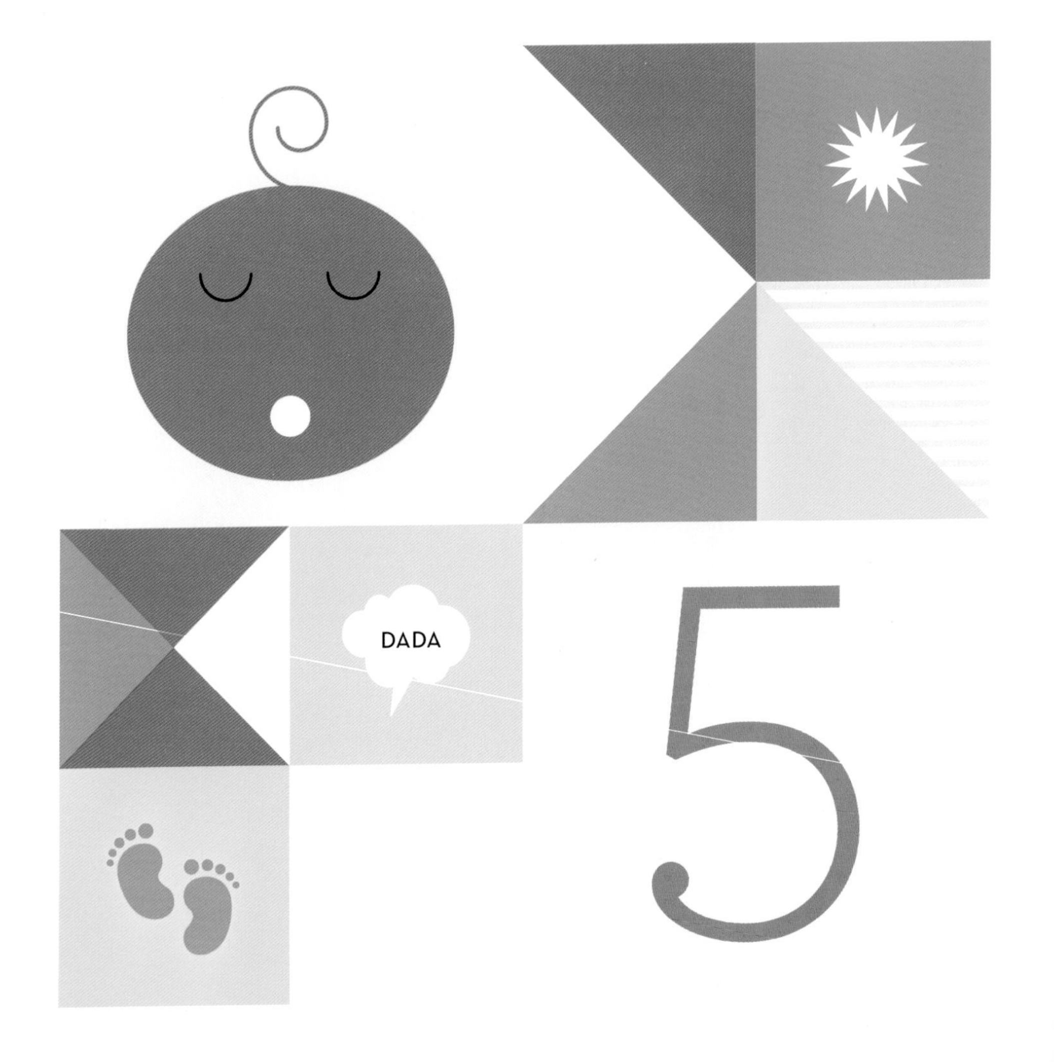
DADA
5

Your Baby Needs Your Help throughout the Hospital Stay

What exactly is the hospital staff going to do with your new baby that may be painful, scary, or both? Here is a rundown of the usual routine procedures and the ways you can make them go a little easier for your little one.

As soon as the baby slides out and the cord is cut, one of two things usually happens. Some medical practitioners place the baby on Mom's abdomen, lay a blanket over the baby, and allow Mom and Dad to enjoy the baby right away. Some hospitals, though, have a policy of placing each new baby on a warming table next to the bed for 10 minutes of observation before the parents can hold the baby.

Actually, you and Mom have the right of choice about this, and Mom will probably appreciate your insisting on immediate tummy time. Besides, the American Academy of Pediatrics, which guides hospital policies regarding newborn care, now states that babies should go straight to the mother's tummy or chest at birth (you can print out this policy from the website www.aap.org).

During the first few minutes after birth, the labor nurse will want to give your baby a thorough exam on the warming table. She will take the baby's vital signs and weight and put identification bracelets on the baby's wrist and ankle. Then she will give the baby a shot of vitamin K in the thigh to prevent bleeding problems. This will obviously sting a little, but will be over quickly. The nurse will also put antibiotic ointment into the baby's eyes to prevent infection. This doesn't hurt, but it will blur the baby's vision until the ointment soaks in. Now, the nurse may take 10 to 15 minutes to go through her routine, including noting all her procedures and findings in the chart. This may sound like a short time, but for the new mom who has just spent hours getting the baby out, this wait can seem like an eternity.

Here's a better scenario: You ask the nurse to leave your baby on Mom's chest for a while. There's no harm in delaying some of the routine procedures up to an hour. While Mom holds the baby, the nurse can get a good enough look to tell if everything seems OK. During this time your baby will probably have her first meal, which the American Academy of Pediatrics says should happen before any medical procedures are performed. After you and Mom enjoy getting to know your baby for a little while, and your baby has a chance to gaze at you both through clear eyes, you invite the nurse to carry out her more thorough assessment.

If your baby is delivered by cesarean-section, this scene will take place in the operating room. The baby will need to be placed on the warming table right away, since Mom's abdomen will be slightly indisposed. But you can stand at your baby's side. After a minute or two, when the baby is kicking and screaming just fine, step up to the table and place your hands on your new baby. When the nurse gives you the OK, pick your baby up and sit with her by Mom's head so Mom can have a look at her and touch her.

Here's what Dr. Bob observes when he attends C-section births:

"Often the new dad isn't sure whether or not he can touch his new baby on the exam table. I grab Dad's hand and pull him into the fray. I love to see the surprise in the dad's eyes as he experiences these first moments."

If your baby needs to be taken to the nursery for any reason while the O.B. finishes the surgery, we suggest you follow your baby so that she can rest in your arms instead of being left alone in a bassinet.

Some babies, such as those born to diabetic mothers and those over nine pounds at birth, require several blood tests in the first few hours. These are usually done by pricking the heel to get out a few drops of blood. Some nurses like to take the baby to the nursery for these tests, but they can be just as easily accomplished in your room. If you don't want the baby to leave your sight or Mom's side, speak up. If the nurse insists that what she needs to do can only be done in the nursery, go with your baby.

The first bath is another procedure that can be delayed. Babies come out with a white creamy substance called vernix on the skin. This natural coating moisturizes and protects a baby's sensitive skin. But nurses don't like goopy babies, so they may offer to give your baby an immediate, thorough scrub-down in the nursery. If you've ever seen a newborn get a bath, you know that they scream and shiver the whole time. It's not pleasant. There's no good reason to give Baby a bath during this first day. Enjoy some quiet time, get some sleep together, and let your baby nurse a few times. *Then* you and your mate can give your baby a gentle sponge bath right on Mom's bed.

Before your baby goes home, she will get a blood screening test for PKU (phenylketonuria) and other rare disorders. It can take several minutes to get the required number of drops of blood out of your baby's heel for this test, so be ready with your finger. Here's another hint: Ask the nurse to warm the baby's heel with a warm wet washcloth for several minutes before the test. This will get the blood flowing better and shorten the procedure.

The baby may get a hearing test as well. This painless evaluation may be done in the nursery (you should insist on tagging along) or in your room.

If your baby boy is going to have a circumcision (a topic we cover in the next chapter), this should be done a day or two after he is born. Again, feel free to tag along for moral support. You can either get right up next to your baby and let him suck on your finger for comfort, or you can stand back or sit across the room and mentally project peaceful thoughts to him.

Whenever your baby wakes during the night, go and get the nurse to check on both the baby and her mother. Then ask the nurse to give you three to four hours without interruption. Tell her that you will buzz her when the baby wakes up again so she won't have to wake all three of you.

A hospital is probably the hardest place in the world to get a good night's sleep. As soon as you get the baby fed, changed, and off to sleep, and you think that you can finally get a few hours of much-needed shut-eye, you'll hear a knock on the door. In comes someone to take your wife's and baby's vital signs and ask how everything is going. "Everything was fine until now," you may be tempted to say. Now the baby is crying and nobody is sleeping. The worst part is that this scene will repeat every two hours all night.

Here's how you can help: Whenever your baby wakes during the night, go and get the nurse to check on both the baby and her mother. Then ask the nurse to give you three to four hours without interruption. Tell her that you will buzz her when the baby wakes up again so she won't have to wake all three of you. If you are the only dad on the floor with this request, it shouldn't be a problem for her. (Don't spread this idea to other dads until *your* wife and baby are ready for discharge.)

Some dads are so tired after their long ordeal of childbirth that they go home to get some sleep, leaving Mom and the baby in the hospital. We can understand this when there are other kids at home. But if the idea of running home to sleep enters your mind after the birth of your first child, we trust you will keep it to yourself. Do not ask your partner if she minds. Just asking will take away all the points you gained from standing by her side through childbirth. Besides, if you leave, no one will be there to run interference for your baby and her mom. So, get comfortable on that floor mat or narrow cot. It's only for a night or two.

Some hospitals will try to convince you to put your baby in the nursery overnight so you and Mom can get some rest. Other hospitals insist that you care for the baby the whole time in your room. Some don't even have nurseries anymore. We recommend you keep the baby with you. Babies who go to the nursery generally spend time crying, even screaming, if there aren't enough nurses' arms to go around. Also, in the nursery your breastfed baby would likely get a bottle of formula or a pacifier while you sleep. This could interfere with her learning to latch on to the breast correctly. Again, the American Academy of Pediatrics can be your best defense: Its policy clearly states that breastfed babies should not receive bottles or pacifiers.

Here's something every new breastfeeding mom and her mate should know: It takes three to five days for Mom's milk to come in. Until then the breasts make a very rich fluid called colostrum, but it comes out in very small quantities. By day two, your baby is going to get hungry. Mom should nurse her every two hours, or more if she wants, to keep the baby content and to help her milk to come in faster. Don't worry if sometimes the baby won't wake up and feed after two hours. Wait an hour and try again. You may notice that by day three your baby's hunger will have increased, and if Mom's milk isn't flowing yet, your baby will express her displeasure clearly. If Mom keeps up the frequent nursing, though, her milk will soon come in and fill up that hungry tummy.

Does the baby need formula in these first few days? No, she doesn't. Babies are born with a lot of extra water inside to keep them hydrated for a few days until the milk comes. Will a nurse try to convince you to give the baby some formula anyway? Possibly.

She may tell you that your baby will get dehydrated. In most cases this simply isn't true, and saying it can cause unnecessary worry for a new mom. Keep encouraging Mom to satisfy the baby at the breast, and by day four she'll have plenty of milk.

If you haven't already, you and your mate can put all your preferences for your birth and hospital stay onto paper before you go to the hospital. Upon admission to the hospital, show this "birth plan" to the O.B. or midwife and the nurse who will care for the mom and baby. Even better, go over your preferences with your medical practitioner at a prenatal visit or with a labor-and-delivery nurse during your prenatal tour of the hospital.

We've given you a lot of warnings about hospitals, but we don't mean to paint them in a negative light. Actually, hospital nurses are a great help to new parents. Sometimes hospital policies and procedures interfere with the natural bonding between parents and their baby. We simply want you to be aware of what your options are and how to look out for the well-being of the new mom and baby. Be courteous with the hospital staff; they are there to help. But don't be afraid to ask questions and stand up for your baby.

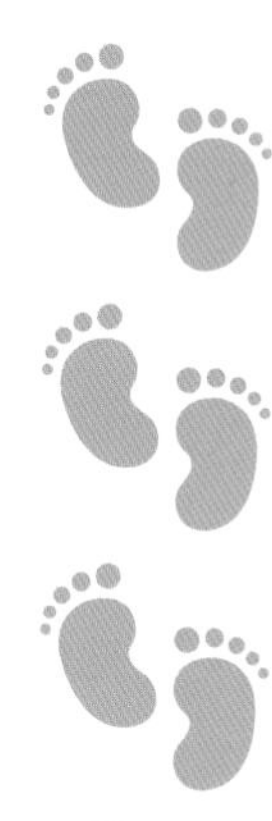

One way to smooth over any friction between you and the hospital staff is to ask one of your visiting friends or family members to bring in a plate of homemade cookies or a similar treat. Take the dish to the nurses' station as a way of saying, "Thank you for all your wonderful help." This will immediately get you known as "the couple in 287 who brought the cookies" instead of "that high-maintenance couple down the hall."

DADA
6

You'll Have to Make a Decision about Circumcision

Before you leave the hospital, there's one thing you need to decide if you have a boy. Years ago, almost all American boys were circumcised. These days, many parents struggle with the circumcision decision, and many are choosing to leave the foreskin intact. Often a mom does not want her son circumcised, but the dad does. In our experience, many moms leave the decision up to Dad. When making your decision, you may encounter many misconceptions and out-of-date information. Here is a summary of the pertinent facts you should consider.

There are no significant medical benefits to routine circumcision, according to the American Academy of Pediatrics. It used to be thought that circumcised men had a much lower chance of penile cancer and that their long-term sexual partners had a lower chance of cervical cancer. We now know that these benefits are minimal. Intact foreskins occasionally get red and swollen from minor infections, but these are easily treated with warm soaks and washing. Worse infections are rare and easily treated with antibiotics. Even if every uncircumcised man got one or two such infections in the course of his life, this would not be a good reason to circumcise at birth. Very rarely, a boy or man will have recurring foreskin infections that necessitate a surgical circumcision, and in this case he might regret that he was not circumcised at birth. Again, though, frequent infections are very rare. We also used to think that circumcised boys and men had a much lower chance of bladder infections, but in fact the difference in risk is very small and exists only for the first few years of life. After that, circumcised boys and men are just as likely to get bladder infections as uncircumcised men. Your decision whether to circumcise should be based on factors apart from any potential medical benefits.

What are some of the nonmedical reasons to consider circumcision? Some people circumcise in accordance with a religious or cultural tradition. Others do it so the baby will look like Dad. In reality, the main difference your child will notice between your penis and his is the hair. Dr. Jim learned this when his son was five:

"I was walking through a mall with Jonathan when we happened upon some acquaintances of mine. As I was introducing

him, Jonathan exclaimed, 'My dad has a hairy penis!' I wanted to sink through the floor."

Other parents worry about locker-room teasing, but today uncircumcised schoolkids are in good company. Fewer and fewer people in the United States are circumcising their boys. (When Dr. Jim was in junior high, there was only one uncircumcised boy in the locker room, but since he happened to be the best player on the soccer team there was no teasing even then.) Currently, around half of the infant males in the United States are being left intact, up from 23 percent in the early 1980s. Most countries in Europe and the rest of the world do not routinely circumcise.

Finally, some parents worry that an uncircumcised penis is too much trouble to clean, especially during childhood. It is true that the foreskin collects white stuff underneath, but this just means there is one more area to wash in the shower. And since you should not pull back the foreskin until it retracts naturally between three years of age and adolescence, there is nothing to clean until then. (If you try to pull the foreskin back before it is ready, your baby will protest loudly, and you could cause irritation or infection.) Over time, the foreskin will loosen by itself and the glans will slowly be revealed. Once it retracts easily, pulling it back and cleaning it during a bath becomes a part of regular hygiene.

Many parents have shared with us their reasons for not circumcising. Some just want to leave nature alone. Whether they believe that God created foreskins or that men evolved with them, these parents can't see a reason to change what nature has provided.

Other parents understand that the foreskin serves some biological purposes: It is filled with nerves and is extremely sensitive to touch. It also protects the glans from the constant rubbing and chafing against clothing that could desensitize it over the years. This preserves sexual pleasure (although one circumcised dad told us, "If I had any *more* sensation there, I wouldn't be able to last long enough to please my wife"). There are also some ethical issues to consider. Some individuals and groups, including some medical societies, oppose routine circumcision because they feel it is unethical for a parent to alter a child's penis without the child's consent. Some circumcised men have expressed anger over their plight.

Some parents worry that the circumcision will be traumatically painful for their baby. Fortunately, most doctors inject an anesthetic around the penis to numb it, so babies usually don't feel any pain during the procedure (although the penis will be somewhat sore for about a week). Babies often just lie there calmly looking around, sucking on a pacifier or a parent's finger. Some even fall asleep. But circumcision is not always peaceful. Some babies scream through the whole procedure, even if they are anesthetized. Some doctors use no anesthesia, which can make the ordeal traumatic.

Parents sometimes choose to wait until their babies are a week or two old before having them circumcised. These babies often cry more through the whole procedure, even with anesthesia. It seems that older babies are more aware of what is going on, and they hate being strapped down. Babies seem to be calmer during circumcision when it is done in the hospital on the second or third day after birth. If you decide to have your boy circumcised, we think the sooner the better.

Most parents feel that as soon as their baby is circumcised his penis will become "maintenance free." This is far from the truth. You will have to put petroleum jelly over the sore penis with every diaper change for about a week. And your job doesn't end there. It is common for the raw edge of the cut skin to restick to the head of the penis. You should make sure your doctor checks for such an adhesion and unsticks it at the one- or two-month checkup. This may hurt a little bit.

When our sons were born, we decided not to decide about their foreskins. We figured that if they wanted to get circumcised later on, they could. It turned out that one of Dr. Bob's kids needed a circumcision along with bladder surgery at age two because of recurring bladder infections. There were no regrets about not circumcising the boy as a newborn; he would have needed the bladder surgery either way. As for the other boys, they will make a lot of decisions about their bodies as they get older—whether to get tattoos, whether to get piercings . . . and whether to keep their foreskins. Some men today wish they still had their foreskins. Many are glad they were circumcised. We figured we'd just let our kids decide for themselves.

If you are going to circumcise your baby, you should feel certain about your decision. If you are unsure, don't rush to have it done in the hospital just to get it over with. Live with your baby's intact penis for a few weeks. Then, if you are sure about circumcising, your pediatrician can do it in the office at any time in the baby's first six weeks of life.

DADA
7

You Are Part of the Breastfeeding Team

Many new dads feel there are certain things they can't do quite as well as moms can, and most moms would probably agree. We prefer to say that dads tend to do things a little differently sometimes. Not worse, not better. Just different. But there is one thing that even we have to admit we're just no good at, and that's breastfeeding. When men realize we are no good at something, we often shrug the thing off as unimportant anyway. In this case, nothing could be further from the truth. Not only is breastfeeding important, but your role in supporting the breastfeeding mom is a crucial one. Here is why.

Breastfeeding doesn't always come automatically for a new mom and baby. They have to work at it. The baby may not latch on correctly. Mom's nipples may feel sore. Still, with help from another mom or breastfeeding consultant and with encouragement from you, there is almost nothing that need stand in the way of a successful breastfeeding relationship.

Nothing can drain a new mom's confidence, however, more than a husband who doesn't understand the importance of breastfeeding. We've heard dads say things like this: "Let's just give up—it's so much work." "We'll just use formula, honey." "You're exhausted and aren't making enough milk." "Bottles will be so much easier."

Contrast this lack of support with the more encouraging words we've heard from other dads: "Let's keep working at this together. You can do it." "I know you are tired and this is challenging, but formula just isn't as good." "I'll help you do whatever it takes to successfully breastfeed our baby."

Often men like to find quick solutions to problems. But most women, our wives tell us, don't like to hear quick answers; they want to know that their husbands understand the challenge and are there for support. Be ready with words of encouragement—your mate is going to need them.

You may be wondering what is so special about breastfeeding. Why does it even matter? There are hundreds of reasons, but perhaps knowing a few will help spur your support of your mate's breastfeeding relationship with your baby. Breastfeeding is good for a baby's health. Breastfed babies have a lower incidence of allergies and asthma and are also less likely to contract a variety of illnesses. Breastfeeding also helps protect babies from SIDS (Sudden Infant Death Syndrome). Children and adults who were breastfed as infants are less likely to experience cancer or diabetes. Finally, breastfeeding is good for a woman's health. Women who breastfeed a baby for a year or more significantly decrease their own risks of breast and ovarian cancer, especially if either of these cancers run in the family.

Breast milk doesn't just protect your baby from illness. It actually builds a better brain. Breastfed babies develop higher IQs; in fact, the longer they are breastfed, the higher their intelligence. A baby's brain forms new nerve connections every day during the first few years of life, and breast milk has specific growth factors that promote these connections. It's as if the baby's brain is a huge home entertainment system with a million wires, only a few of which are hooked up at first. Every day a few more wires get plugged in, until after a few years the whole system is fully functional. Breast milk ensures that all the wires get plugged into the right spots. The brain of a formula-fed baby doesn't form as many connections. This is one reason that breastfeeding should continue for at least one year; two years is even better.

Besides the advantages for Mom and Baby, does breastfeeding offer any advantages for dads? You bet. You'll sleep better if your baby isn't awake all night coughing and sniffling. You'll save

Breast milk doesn't just protect your baby from illness. It actually builds a better brain. Breastfed babies develop higher IQs; in fact, the longer they are breastfed, the higher their intelligence.

thousands of dollars in doctor's bills and formula costs. Dr. Bob discovered an extra perk:

"I got to sleep the whole night through! Our babies usually woke up hungry a couple of times each night (OK, sometimes five or six, my wife informs me), and my wife quickly learned how useless I was getting them back to sleep. So I was off the hook for night duty. I slept so well that each morning I would have to ask my wife how the night went.

"I remember waking up one morning to find my six-month-old sitting up in bed next to me staring at my chest. He leaned in close, opened up his mouth, and tried to get his jaws on me. I laughed so loudly he never tried it again."

As dads, are we completely useless when it comes to breastfeeding? We don't have to be. Here's how you can help. In the early weeks, a mom needs a couple of extra hands in getting the baby positioned for nursing. Ask how you can help with setup for each feeding. Breastfeeding can put a strain on Mom's back, so be ready to give her a massage each night. Nursing a baby will make Mom thirsty, so be her water boy; keep several water bottles filled and placed throughout the house. Healthy snacks are a must for nursing moms, so keep bowls of trail mix, fresh fruit, dried fruit, nuts, wholesome crackers, and anything else she likes within easy reach.

Dr. Jim kept a stack of pillows next to the bed:

"For the first few weeks of middle-of-the-night feedings, my wife would need several pillows to support her back and arms. It

was my job to help her get comfortable; I could go back to sleep once she was propped up in feeding position. Luckily, she soon learned how to nurse while lying on her side."

We often hear dads say they feel a little left out because they can't feed the baby. Don't pressure your mate into letting you give a bottle; most women feel that the trouble of pumping isn't worth the little break they get by letting Dad feed the baby. And be warned: If Mom does let you give a daytime bottle, she may recruit you for a night shift as well. You shouldn't ask to give a bottle at all during the first month; wait until breastfeeding is off to a solid start. And don't offer a pacifier in the first few weeks. Both pacifiers and bottle nipples can confuse a baby and disrupt breastfeeding.

Even after the first month, there can be drawbacks to giving a breastfed baby an occasional bottle. Some babies begin to prefer the bottle and start to fight the breast. If Mom skips feedings to let you give the baby a bottle, she may experience problems with her milk supply. These problems can lead to a downward spiral that results in early weaning.

What can you do when breastfeeding isn't getting off to a smooth start? Start by holding your baby while Mom calls La Leche League. This is an international support group of breast-feeding mothers who volunteer to help new moms over the phone. La Leche's toll-free number is 877-4- LaLeche (877-452-5324). If a La Leche leader can't solve the problem, help Mom track down a certified lactation consultant (who puts the letters IBCLC after her name). A lactation consultant will spend hours with the mom and baby, if needed, until the two of them get it right. This service will cost money, but your insurance company may reimburse you if you get a note from the baby's doctor. You may be able to use a hospital-employed lactation consultant at low cost. A lactation consultant could turn out to be the most important medical professional in the new mom and baby's life, even more important than a pediatrician. Not calling a lactation consultant when feeding isn't going well is like not calling a doctor when you're having severe chest pains. Make the investment in your baby's nutrition and health. Do whatever it takes to help your baby and Mom succeed at life's most important first step.

DADA
8

You Can Ace Baby 101

So far you've learned the basics of welcoming your newborn into the world. You've held your baby, changed a diaper or two, and become your wife's water boy, massage therapist, and snack-bar attendant. Now what? Most things in life come with clear directions. You get a new job, and you start meeting goals and deadlines. You buy a car, and you start driving it. You buy a new home entertainment system, you set it up and enjoy! But exactly what are new dads supposed to do with a new baby?

We already offered the theory that there's only one thing you really have to do—hold him. But that's only half the story. Babies also need to be changed, burped, bathed, and dressed, over and over, and who's going to do all that? "The baby's mother," you may say. Wrong. One of the best ways you can shine as a dad is to jump in and do your share of all the little things that add up to a lot. Every task you do brings you a little closer to your baby.

Many new dads are very unsure about how to physically handle a new baby. A few have actually asked us if it was OK to touch the baby. Dr. Jim recently heard a new dad say that he learned a lot from seeing how the nurses handled his baby:

"Watching the nurse give the baby his first bath, he was quite surprised at how much the baby was getting squeezed and rubbed. The bath wasn't exactly rough, but it didn't seem very gentle. After realizing that his new baby was not made of eggshells, Dad had much more confidence in carrying him around, changing his diaper, and swaddling him. He no longer worried that the baby would break."

We have discussed how useless you may feel at feeding time (unless your baby is bottle-fed), but you can certainly come in handy when the feeding is done. Offer to burp the little guy after he nurses. How do you do this? There are two basic methods: Either hold your baby upright with his tummy pressed against your shoulder, or sit him on your lap and press his tummy with the heel of your hand. In either position, firmly pat the baby's upper and

One of the best ways you can shine as a dad is to jump in and do your share of all the little things that add up to a lot. Every task you do brings you a little closer to your baby.

middle back with the flat of your hand until the job is done.

Oops. Did we forget to mention that you need to place a spit-up rag over your shoulder or on your lap? Sorry about that warm ooze dripping down your back. The burp rag is supposed to catch that. Now you know.

If you don't get a burp within a minute or so, change positions. If you still get nothing, don't just hand the baby over to his mom without warning her, or half his lunch is going to come up all over her new outfit. Then who do you think is in trouble? Not the baby, that's for sure. If your baby just won't let it out, wait for a few minutes, then try again. Usually this will get you what you want. Don't worry if the first few times your wife rolls her eyes, grabs the baby, and with one tap elicits a prize-winning belch. You'll get better at it with practice.

Dr. Bob recalls his first burping experience with baby number three:

"I remember the baby was fussy that first night. We couldn't figure it out. He had been fed, changed, held, and bounced, but he wouldn't stop crying. After my wife and I passed him back and forth for an hour, I put him over my shoulder, and out it came: Burrrrp. Oh, yeah, I thought, we forgot to burp him after he ate. Actually, my wife forgot to burp him. I saved the day."

Another way you can really shine is in diapering. Wait! If your baby is only a day or two old, before you undo that diaper, we must warn you: These first few diaper changes are not the usual

cute, soft, yellow baby poops. No, no, no. For the first couple of days, the diapers will be filled with black, tarry, sticky muck called meconium (Latin for "whoa, what a mess"). This is the stuff that has been sitting in the gut for weeks and weeks, and the first few diapers will probably be the messiest you'll ever see. Babies often poop during or right after feeding, so Mom will probably appreciate the five-minute break if you take over. Grab a diaper, diaper cream, and a new outfit in case the diaper has leaked. Have three or four baby wipes out of the box and ready. Lay your baby on a changing pad, either on the floor or on a changing table (we suggest the floor, since squirmy babies have been known to roll off even the most secure changing tables). Position the new diaper underneath your baby's bottom. Remove the front of the dirty diaper, and use it to wipe most of the mess off the baby. Then fold the diaper underneath the baby. Use the wipes to clean off the rest. Be sure to get it all, or else Mom may blame the resulting diaper rash on you. Remove the dirty diaper and position the new diaper underneath the baby (with a disposable diaper, the tape tabs go in the back). Slather on plenty of diaper cream (again, to avoid getting blamed for a rash). Then tape on the new diaper (or Velcro, snap, or pin it on if using cloth diapers). Tape the folded dirty diaper closed so it won't smell up the trash. Above all, avoid getting any mess on the changing pad. "But isn't that what it's there for?" you may wonder. Yes, but then somebody has to wash the changing pad.

For wet diapers you do everything the same; the job just isn't as messy. For girl babies, rinse the soap out of the baby wipes with warm water (or use a wet cloth) for the first few weeks to avoid irritation. One more thing: If you have a boy, don't ever look away from that little penis while it's uncovered. As you change the diaper, your baby is watching you intently, just waiting for you to turn your head so he can pee all over you. You'll know the little guy is about to let loose when his penis sticks straight up. Keep an extra diaper close at hand so you can grab and cover at a moment's notice. The funny thing is, he'll often squirt himself in the face instead of you.

If you really want to look like a diapering pro, try a technique Dr. Jim learned with his son—the ankle grab. If you've ever carried two bottles of beer in one hand, you already know how to do this: Simply grab the baby's ankles together with one hand, and lift them toward his head. This raises his butt, pins his upper body down, and exposes the diaper area. Your other hand is free to do the wiping.

What? You don't like changing diapers? We don't know any dad who enjoys this messy task, but a baby's doody is our duty. One dad we know got out of diaper duty for good by purposely putting the diapers on too loose. After they leaked poop several times, Mom banned him from diaper changing forever. When your baby needs a diaper change, you're free to grab a beer and go watch the football game. And miss out on raising your child.

You may find it useful to know what baby poop is generally supposed to look like. This way, when you see something unusual (because you are changing so many of the dirty diapers, right?) you'll know whether to freak out or relax. As you've already learned, in the first days a baby produces black, sticky meconium. As the baby begins to take in more milk, the stools change to greenish and mucousy. By the end of the first week, they are yellow and seedy-looking (like a mixture of gourmet mustard and yellow cottage cheese). Don't be surprised if the poop occasionally has a different color or consistency. There's no need to ponder this unless the change persists for a few days.

Now, what about that oozing, slimy stump that used to be the umbilical cord? What are you supposed to do with that? For one thing, avoid pulling on it; you don't want to get blamed for your baby's cord coming off too early. Also, don't worry if it oozes some mucus or blood; this is normal. We used to recommend that parents wipe around the cord stump with alcohol several times each day, but research has shown that this may not be necessary. If the stump becomes red, swollen, or foul-smelling, though, you should start applying rubbing alcohol at every other diaper change. Give sponge baths rather than tub baths until the umbilical cord dries up and falls off, between one and four weeks after birth.

How often does a baby need a bath? The truth is, babies don't get dirty, except around the face from milk and spit-up and in the diaper area. These places can usually be kept clean enough with baby wipes and spit-up rags. Babies really need a full bath only once or twice a week. Some parents are fine with that, but others, especially moms, meticulously wash their babies every day. There's no harm in being too clean.

Exactly how do you give a tiny, squirmy, slippery-when-wet baby a bath? It's not easy. We're not going to give you directions. We suggest you just watch Mom a few times, then let her observe you do it, and wait for her OK before you attempt this on your own. Or, if you are both clueless, follow our directions in *The Baby Book: Everything You Need to Know About Your Baby from Birth to Age Two*, by Sears and Sears (Little Brown, 2013).

Let's see, what else can we dads do with a baby? Oh, yeah! Dressing. This takes extreme skill. You've never seen such a confusing array of snaps until you've tried to dress a baby. It can take forever to figure out which snaps go where. You'll spend five minutes snapping on the baby's outfit only to come to the end and find that you are one snap off. Then you have to undo all the snaps to find the missing one.

Here's how to dress a baby in a onesies: Lay the outfit on the floor with all the snaps undone. Lay your baby face up on top of the outfit. Work his arms in first (this is key), then his legs. Put the snaps together starting at each foot and working up to the diaper. Then skip to the neck and snap down to the waist. The last step, the crotch, is the most confusing. Save it for last, and then just snap and resnap as necessary until it looks right.

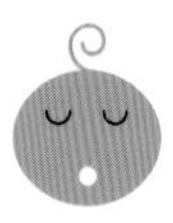

There's nothing that impresses a new mom more than a new dad who can deftly dress a baby in under two minutes with the diaper on securely and all the snaps in the right place.

What about outfits that don't have snaps down the front? They usually have a few snaps on one side of the neck. Undo these, pull the outfit over baby's head, and then work it down around the rest of baby's body. It may look easiest to put the baby leg-first through the neck hole and then pull the outfit up over his body, but this never works. Again, put in the baby's arms before the legs, and then snap up the legs. Don't forget the neck snaps; some moms hate it when these are left undone.

Now why are we wasting time in a manly book for men discussing baby fashion? Because there's nothing that impresses a new mom more than a new dad who can deftly dress a baby in under two minutes with the diaper on securely and all the snaps in the right place. Just thought you'd want to really excel as a new dad.

If your baby isn't being breastfed, you will obviously need to help out with the bottles (if it *wasn't* obvious to you before, take this as a friendly smack on the back of your head). How do you sterilize bottles? How much do you feed the baby? How often? What kind of formula should you use? These are all very good questions, but they are beyond the scope of this book. We invite you to read all about formula feeding in *The Baby Book.*

There are two things a man must never drop: a football and a baby. Dr. Jim has witnessed a few close calls:

"I recently walked into a hospital room to check on a newborn patient, and I saw Dad sitting in the rocking chair, cuddling his new baby. It was nice to see that the two were starting to bond

already. Then Dad gingerly started to hand me the baby so that I could do the first exam, and nearly dropped him. Dad was holding the baby in his elbows, snuggled into his chest—a great position for a nap, but not for a 'hand-off.' Dad's more experienced brother, who was in the room visiting, started laughing and said, 'If your high-school football coach could only see you now! That was almost the biggest fumble of your life!' Dad was being so gentle with his newborn that he almost dropped him.

"I then showed Dad a much more secure way of handling the baby. From the cuddle position, slide your hands in and grab him—just like a football. One hand should be under his bottom with your thumb and forefinger gripping his upper thigh; the other hand should support his upper back and his neck. This technique reminds me of how a quarterback carries the football while running the option play—very securely. You can't drop him this way."

Oh, there's one last thing. During the first few weeks, there are 15 peculiarities every new baby may have. They are completely normal, but they tend to worry new parents. Become very familiar with this list. Then, when your baby does these things and Mom wants to rush him to the doctor, you can calmly and confidently say, "Don't worry, honey. All babies do that. It's normal." You may want to mark the next page for quick reference in case you have to prove you're right when she looks at you as if you're insane.

Hiccups Most babies get these for several minutes after feedings.

Spitting up Some babies seem to bring up their entire lunch after each feeding. As long as Baby seems satisfied, not fussy, and is gaining weight, don't worry. This is a laundry problem, not a medical problem.

Diaper rash Every new baby gets red around the anus as the sensitive bottom gets accustomed to sitting in poop. You may even see a little bit of bleeding. Simply change Baby more often, put on a thick layer of white diaper cream, and he should be fine.

Stuffy nose and congested breathing Most babies get a little stuffy for several weeks. No, your baby probably isn't sick. His nose is just getting used to everything that's in the air he breathes. This too shall pass. Mom can drip breast milk or nasal saline into his nose and suction it out with a bulb syringe to help keep the nose clear.

Rash Many babies get red bumps, pimples, and splotches on the face, neck, and upper body. This normal newborn rash doesn't have a known cause, and it will fade away on its own.

Dry, peeling skin Baby's skin will appear to look dry in the first few days, especially on the extremities. You don't have to use any lotion. The skin isn't actually dry; the outer layer is simply peeling away and the skin underneath is perfectly healthy.

Crusty scalp Called "cradle cap," this harmless condition isn't a reflection of poor hygiene. Rub on some olive oil before each bath to soften the crust, then gently run a comb through to lift it out. The baby's mother may not know this trick yet, so you'll look like a genius.

Gas Every baby passes gas. As long as the gas isn't accompanied by extreme fussing, you can just be proud of your little guy. If the gas often seems painful, ask your doctor for advice.

Sneezing Babies do this a lot in the early weeks. It's not usually a sign of allergies or illness; it's just a baby's way of keeping the nose clear.

Vaginal discharge or bleeding In girls, this is normal for the first week or two.

Red-tinged urine You may see what looks like red brick dust in the diaper. Don't worry; it isn't blood. It will pass in a few days.

Irregular breathing New babies often breathe rapidly for several seconds and then take a long pause. This is normal.

Red splotch in the eye Getting squeezed through the birth canal often causes a red mark in the whites of the eyes. This will go away in a few weeks. If most of the eye is red, your baby's doctor should check it.

Green eye drainage This is fairly common. As long as the eyes are not red, you don't need to worry. Tell Mom to put a few drops of breast milk into each eye after feedings. Yup, breast milk. It cures anything.

Twitching Many babies' arms and legs twitch briefly, especially when falling asleep. This is due to an immature nervous system. Tell the doctor if the twitching ever continues for more than 30 seconds.

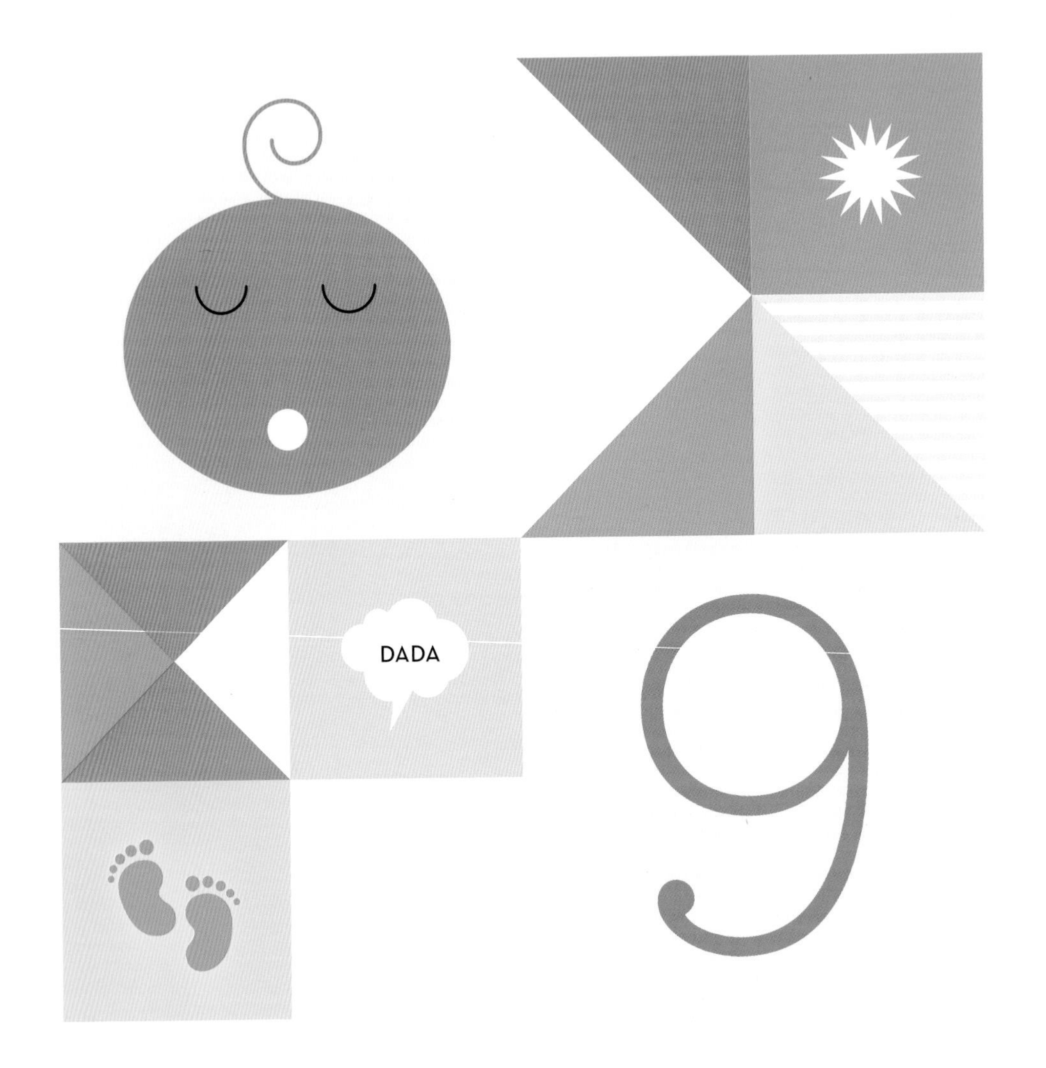
DADA
9

You Can Raise Your Baby (Almost) for Free

There's no such thing as a free lunch, and most people would say there's no such thing as a free baby either. Young couples often tell us, "We're saving up to have a baby," or "We're waiting until we are more financially secure to start having kids." In today's dual-income world, the loss of one salary when a parent stays home can be quite a burden. But we've been pleasantly surprised at just how little babies can cost, at least in the first couple of years. Once they get older, the bills begin to pile up—for food, clothes, toys, school, fun activities. But right now you have just one little baby, and she shouldn't cost you much.

Our first babies were both born while we were in medical school, so we weren't earning any money. Our wives were working while pregnant, but they were both planning to stay at home once the babies were born. So how did we survive? We got extra student loans to live on. We got a little help from our parents. We lived within our means. And we found plenty of ways to *not* spend money on our babies. Here is how you can do it.

First let's talk about what should *not* cost you money.

Baby food, for one thing. For the first six months it's free if it's all breast milk. Mom has to eat more to make that food, but breastfeeding is like a restaurant where kids eat free when accompanied by a paying adult. All breastfeeding costs is a few nursing bras and nursing shirts. And in the second half of the first year most babies eat very little regular food; most of their nutrients still come from breast milk. You don't have to buy expensive baby food; just let your baby nibble on whatever you're eating or mash her some vegetables. During the toddler years it seems most kids barely eat anything. So, don't feel you have an extra mouth to feed just yet.

If you and your wife are passing up manna from heaven and going with formula instead, we hope you've been saving your money. Formula will cost you about $1,500 for the year, not including bottles and the more frequent doctor visits you are likely to make.

But what about baby clothes, toys, bottles, and so on? Don't these cost a bundle? Hey, that's what baby showers are for. In fact, you shouldn't buy any of these things until you've sorted through the loot from a baby shower or two. You're sure to get outfits, blankets, and almost everything else you'll need for the first year. As the nesting instinct kicks in, many moms-to-be browse the baby boutiques toward the end of pregnancy and spend hundreds of dollars on adorable frills and lace. If your mate is eager to do the same, try to gently rein her in.

What about the clothes your friends and relatives don't buy you? "Got any good way to get all those six- to twelve-month outfits for free?" you ask. Well, not really. But you don't have to spend a lot on clothes if you don't want to. Any friend or relative who has a child a year older than yours will be a perfect source for hand-me-downs. If nobody offers you secondhand clothes, and money is tight, you can buy all you need from a thrift store. You can get clothes at a discount if you peruse the sale racks at the right times. Dr. Bob was impressed with his wife's ability to get for $5 something that cost $50 when it came out six months ago.

Now, let's talk about the big-ticket items. If you haven't already furnished a nursery, you need a matching furniture set, right? Then there's the playpen, the high-chair, the video baby monitor, the fancy cradle, the collapsible stroller, and the baby swing. Plus, you'll need one of those convenient car seats that converts into a baby carrier. It will take a couple of months' salary to pay for all these "necessities."

Here's a little secret: You can do without these things. Sure, some are useful, but you have to decide which are necessities and which are not.

First, your baby doesn't need matching furniture. You don't have to spend a fortune at a specialty furniture store. You might shop around for a reasonably priced combination changing table–dresser, because you will need some place to keep your baby's clothes. You might even find one that will convert into a desk later on, when the baby is out of diapers.

"And she needs a crib, right?" you ask. Well, your baby *does* need a place to sleep, but have your baby first before you spend $500 on a crib. You may find she is perfectly content to sleep in an inexpensive bassinet or cradle for a few months. Or she may wind up in your bed and never even need a crib. Dr. Bob bought a crib for his first baby, but he was glad he spent only $50 on it, because it ended up serving as a laundry basket. Dr. Jim's first child slept much better in bed with Mom and Dad, so he and his wife used their crib money on a king-size bed. Your baby may sleep so well in your room that she never sees the inside of her nursery until she is two or three. If your baby outgrows the cradle or bassinet by four months, and hasn't wound up in your bed by then, *then* go out and buy a crib.

As for the playpen, your baby will play just as well on the floor. Couch cushions make a good barrier if you need to keep her contained for a few minutes.

You *will* need a high-chair—when your baby is about six months old. You should have plenty of time to save up.

As for the playpen, your baby will play just as well on the floor. Couch cushions make a good barrier if you need to keep her contained for a few minutes.

Video baby monitor? Let's just say it's a luxury that you really don't need. A simple audio monitor for $20 is perfect for listening for Baby.

As for a stroller, well, you've got arms, don't you? Honestly, strollers are a lot of trouble to lug around town, fold up and down, and park in your living room. Carrying your baby in your arms or in a baby sling is so much easier. You *will* probably need a stroller someday, when your baby gets too big to carry long distances. But by that time you can easily get away with an inexpensive umbrella type instead of the latest SUV model.

This leaves the car seat. Now of course you need a car seat, but we can save you a bunch of money in this department, too. Invest in a convertible car seat that the baby can use rear facing as an infant, then forward facing until the age of four, then as a booster seat until she is eight. Buying only one seat instead of two or three over several years will save you a bundle.

A car seat that doubles as infant carrier and seat not only is outgrown by Baby's first birthday, but it can also be a safety hazard. Many models have been recalled over the years because the handles have broken and babies have fallen out, or because the seat doesn't lock properly into its base when in the car. Parents commonly set a baby in one of these seats on a table or counter, and sometimes the baby is accidentally knocked onto the floor. Babies who are instead set on the floor in a car seat often fall victim to dropped items or spilled drinks. It's much safer to have your baby up against your body in a sling or in your arms.

Dr. Bob doesn't like to see parents carry babies around in these car seats. A person has to bend sideways away from the carrier just to balance it. This looks so awkward. Are people afraid to just carry their babies?

Picture this: You pick up your baby and put her into the carrier seat. You carry her to the car and insert the seat into the base. You drive to the doctor's office. You remove the carrier seat (with the baby in it, of course) and carry it into the doctor's office. You set the baby in the seat on the floor. Your name is called, and you pick up the seat and carry it into the exam room, where, once again, you place it on the floor. The doctor comes into the room and examines your baby in the car seat, or takes her out for a closer look and puts her back. When the visit is done, you pick up the seat, carry it back out to your car, insert it into the base, make sure it's strapped in right, and drive back home. You carry the seat back into the house and set it down on the floor.

Congratulations. You've just spent an entire hour or two taking your baby to the doctor, and you've managed not to touch her even once.

Admittedly, these car seats can be convenient when your baby falls asleep in the car and you want to move her without waking her, as Dr. Jim notes:

"While I was sitting at the coffee shop writing notes for this

book, a car pulled into a parking space in front of me. A new dad got out of the car, opened the door to the back seat, and pulled out his three-month-old daughter, still sleeping in her snap-in seat. He gently pulled down the sun shade to protect her face, and then he carried her across the parking lot to the convenience store. When he returned a few minutes later carrying the baby and a cold six-pack, I stopped him to tell him I was writing about him. It turned out that this dad would take the baby during her weekend naps and run all his errands while Mom got a much-needed break. He had already been to the hardware store, the pharmacy, and the gas station before making the beer stop. The baby had stayed asleep the whole time! I remember doing the same as this dad when my second child was a baby.

"On the other hand, the next week I saw a mom come into the coffee shop with her baby in a baby sling. I watched her give the baby three kisses, two pats on the head, and one rub on the back all in five minutes. So there is a lot to be said for having your baby in-arms instead of in-seat."

If you have one of these car seats, feel free to use it as a carrier while your baby sleeps, but when she wakes up and wants to see the world with you, leave the seat in the car and use your arms or a baby sling instead.

So, what else is going to cost money? Oh, yeah—medical insurance. Thankfully, adding your baby to your current medical plan will probably cost only a bit more than you are paying now.

We've mentioned many items you don't necessarily need, but there's one thing you really can't do without—diapers. And, yes, they can be quite expensive. You can certainly save money by buying in bulk from a warehouse store. But if you need to pinch pennies, use cloth diapers. If you can't find them in stores, you can order them easily online. Unfortunately, diaper-washing services aren't as common as they used to be. But by laundering cloth diapers, you will save a "load" of money instead of "wasting" it all on disposables.

So there you have it. Your baby is practically cost-free. Well, at least you don't have to get a second job or sell your baseball-card collection. So don't let the supposed financial burden of a new baby cause you undue stress just yet. There will be plenty of time to worry about money when you have to start paying for Baby's college education.

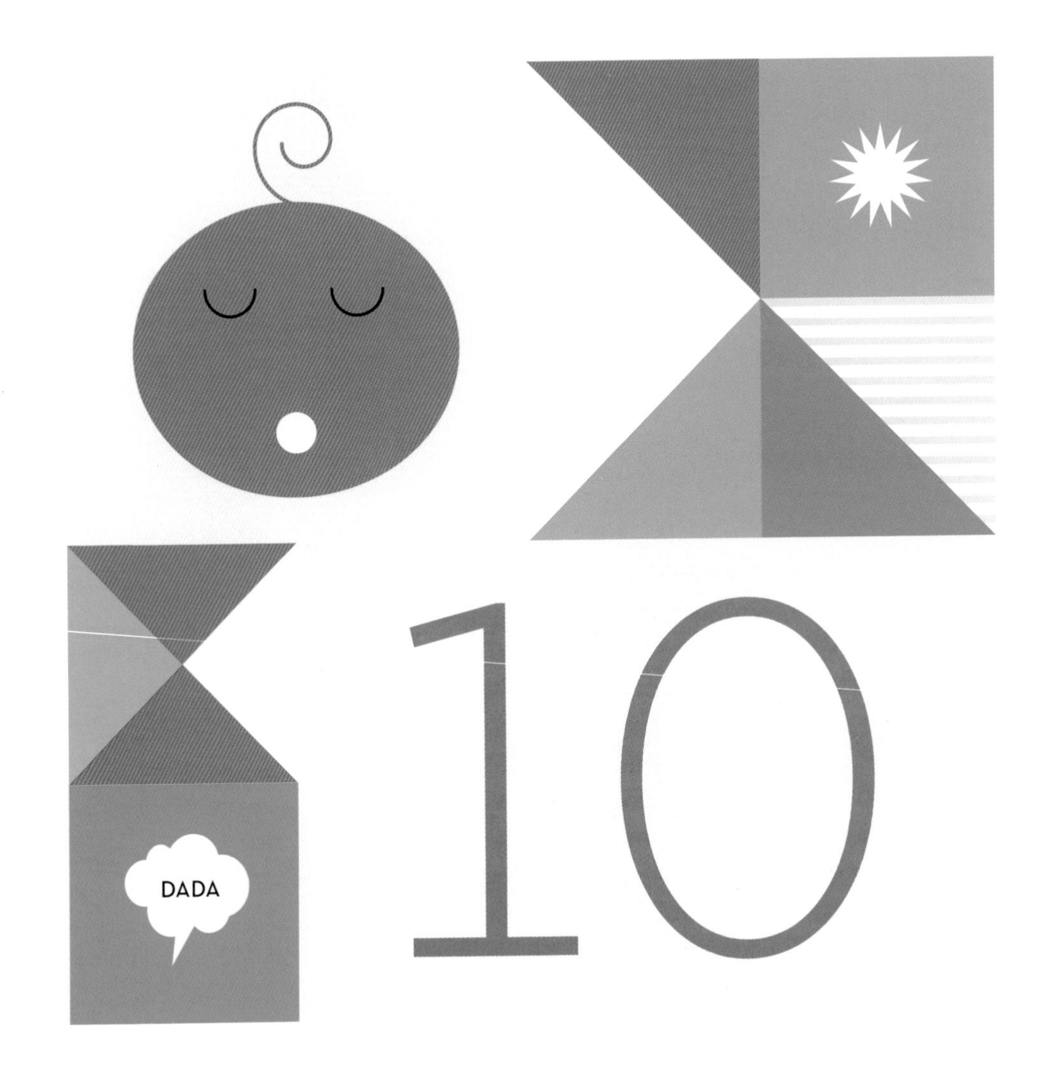
DADA
10

You Can Learn to Speak Baby

Wouldn't it be so much easier if babies could just talk? "Hey, Mom, I'm hungry!" "Hey, Dad, your turn to change my diaper!" "Hey, I'm awake again, and I'm kind of scared. Can someone please come pick me up?" "Ow, my tummy's really hurting. Can you please do something?"

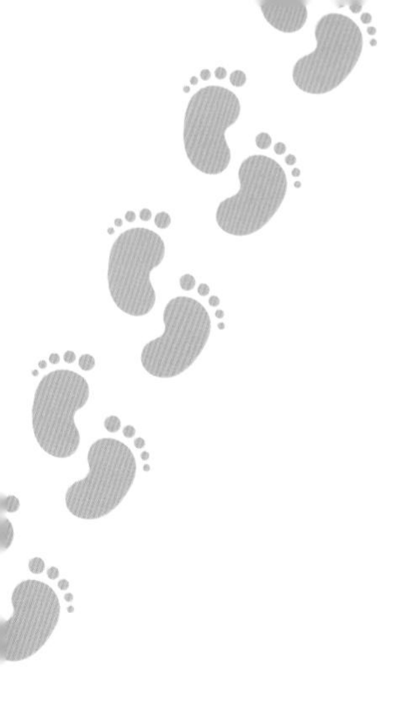

Believe it or not, babies do talk, every day. The problem is, to new parents everything a baby says sounds like "Waaaaaaaaaaaa!"

"Wait a minute," you say. "A cry is just a cry, isn't it? Babies cry when they want something. But this isn't language; it's just an instinctive noise they make, right?" Our experience with five kids of our own and many families in the office suggests otherwise. A baby's cry has different tones, intensities, volumes, and other characteristics that vary according to his needs. Add to that some very obvious body language and facial expressions, and even the most unobservant parent can begin to translate a baby's cries into words.

We enjoy observing parents when a baby cries during an office visit. Dad will say, "I think he's hungry. That's his hunger cry." Mom will reply, "No, that's his poopy diaper cry." Who do we usually think is right? Since this is a book about how wonderful dads can be, we'll leave the answer up to you (with a wink to Mom).

Moms have a translational advantage. The mothering hormone, prolactin, is like a Baby-English dictionary. We dads need to work a little harder, but with practice (and a lot of holding and bonding) we too can learn to speak Baby.

Learning to understand your baby's cries is important, but you must also decide what you are going to do about them. To respond or not to respond? To "spoil" or not to spoil? To be or not to be a dad who believes his baby's cries should be answered in a sensitive and interactive way?

There are two schools of thought on this question. Some people believe that you shouldn't always respond to a baby's cries. Sure, you should be a responsible parent who meets his child's basic needs, and who *usually* tends to the baby when he cries. But sometimes a baby's cries should go unanswered so he doesn't become too dependent. He needs to learn that you won't always be there for him and that sometimes he needs to work things out by himself. He needs to learn that he can't always manipulate you with his cry.

Other people feel that a baby's cries should be answered every time. Young babies don't understand how to manipulate a person; they cry simply to communicate and get their needs met. If you make a baby feel completely secure, if you teach him that he is important to you and that you will always be there for him, he will develop self-confidence and a healthier kind of independence, rooted in a secure foundation.

So, who is right? This is not so much an issue of right and wrong but a question of what type of parent-child relationship you want to have, not only now but also when your baby grows up. Virtually every research study done on this subject has come to the same conclusion: Babies who are more securely attached to their parents and who are less often left to cry by themselves become more independent and emotionally stable as older children, with fewer behavioral and psychological problems. A secure, dependent baby becomes a secure, independent child. A less attached, independent baby may become an insecure, more dependent child. Almost no study has concluded otherwise. So why do people worry about spoiling a baby by holding him too much and never leaving him to cry? Because they read the advice of writers who haven't consulted the research.

But forget what the research shows for a minute. Let's talk about you again. What type of relationship do you want with your baby? Can you go wrong by growing too close to your child? When your baby calls for you, can you truly ever be wrong to respond? If your responsiveness makes your baby want to spend more time with you, is this a bad thing? Or might you instead go wrong by being too detached and distant from your baby?

We believe that the more you treat your baby's cries as language, and the more you respond to this language, the better your baby will become at communicating with you. He will learn to cry less and talk more, using body language as well as sounds. He will learn he doesn't have to cry, because you will be there soon.

Think about what kind of dad you want to be when your kids are a bit older. Are you sometimes going to ignore them when they speak to you? If your five-year-old calls to you, "Dad! I'm cold and scared. Can you pick me up?" are you going to sit there and ignore him so he becomes independent? If this is what you want, then you might as well start ignoring your baby now so he doesn't come to expect too much closeness.

If you really aren't sure how responsive you want to be when your baby cries, try it both ways. Forget everything you've read, and just contemplate how you feel when the baby cries for a few minutes. Do you feel that you should pick the baby up, or do you feel that he can go it alone? Now, if Mom is around, the decision isn't yours alone. Observe your mate—she has the benefit of the mothering hormone, after all. Does she pick the baby up every time he cries? Ask her why she does or doesn't. Talk about it. What do her instincts tell her, and what do yours tell you?

If you trust your own intuition, you'll be right 99 percent of the time. That is enough in any walk of life.

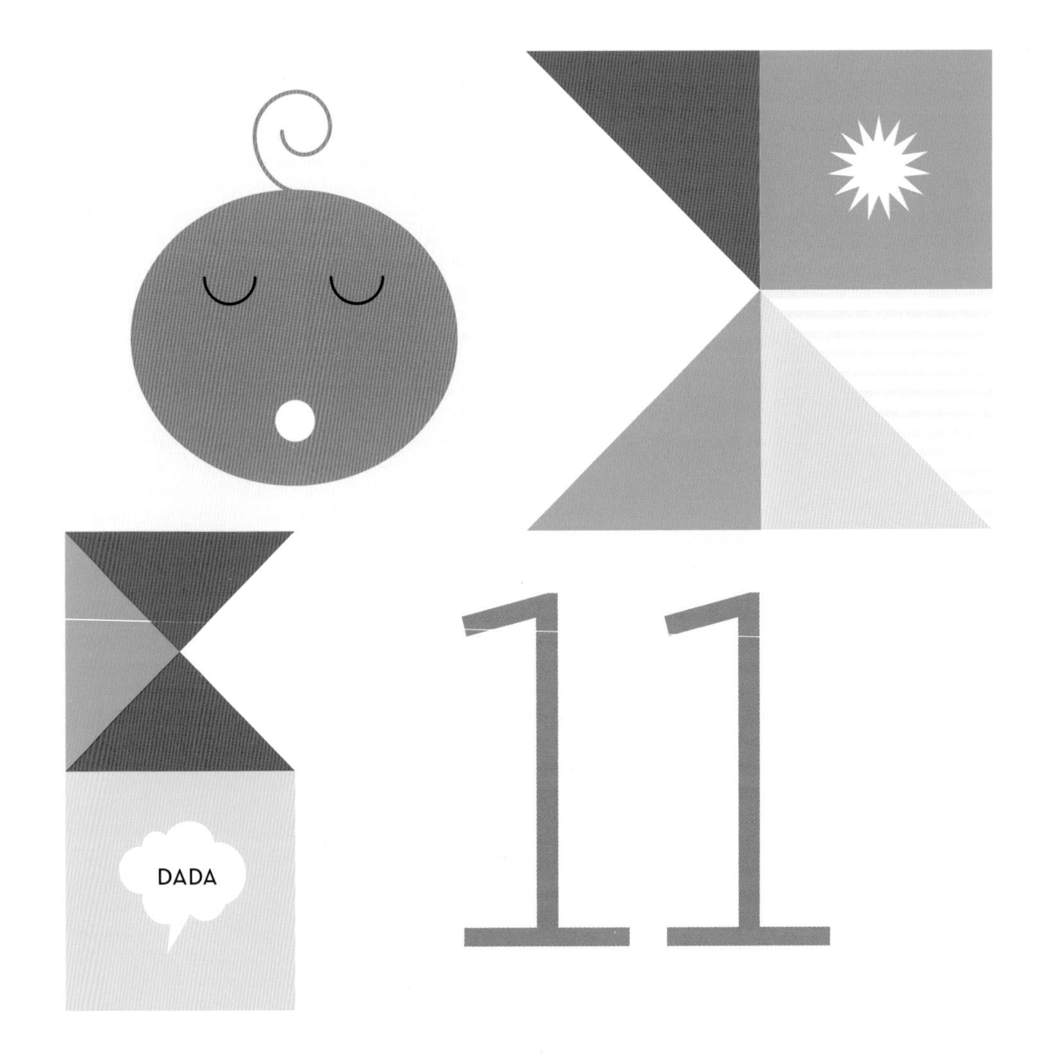
DADA
11

Some Babies Need More

As you drive home from work, you pass by the neighbors' house. They have just had a baby, too, and you see them relaxing on the front porch swing, sipping lemonade and goo-goo-ing at their smiling little baby. You pull the car into your driveway. The porch is empty. In place of a swing are a few dead plants and mud from last month's rain. You turn the engine off and enjoy a moment of peace and quiet.

Then you take a deep breath, step out of the car, and open the house door into chaos. The baby is screaming while Mom dances around the kitchen, bouncing the baby over her shoulder. You look around, hoping to see a glass of lemonade at least. Mom practically tosses the baby into your arms, then collapses onto the couch. You don't smell dinner cooking. You bet the neighbors are enjoying a nice home-cooked meal right now. The baby takes one brief look at you and begins wailing anew.

If this describes your evenings, we sympathize. If you are instead that neighbor with the perfect, happy baby, then you can skip this chapter. Better yet, put down your lemonade and go offer to help your less fortunate friend.

If you have been blessed with a fussy baby, you are probably wondering why your baby cries every time you put her down. Why does the slobber hit the fan every single evening, when happy hour turns into three hours of crying? Why does your baby seem to *need* so much more than most babies you've heard about? Why can't you and your wife sit out on the porch with your lemonade and enjoy the sunset with a happy baby?

Every baby is born with a particular temperament. While some babies are happy to be left alone until they are hungry, others need constant attention. Some seem oblivious to what's going on around them, but others fuss at the slightest disruption. Some couldn't care less whether they are held or not, and others insist on staying glued to a parent 24/7. A baby's temperament changes slightly over the months and years in response to how she is cared for, but in general temperament is determined genetically, before birth. We call babies who are very demanding *high-need babies.*

Some babies are frequent criers not just because of temperament but because they have colic. Here's how you can tell the difference: A colicky baby cries on and off throughout the day no matter what you do to console her. She may scream full-steam for hours on end. Something seems to be hurting her little tummy, and all the holding and bouncing and rocking and sucking in the world makes little difference. A high-need baby, on the other hand, will be perfectly happy as long as her needs are met. What are those needs? Sucking and holding and rocking and bouncing. The minute you put the baby down, she cries. If you try to make her sleep alone, she wakes up and cries. If you try to make her cry it out, she'll scream forever.

So which kind of baby do you have? If you have a baby with colic, the good news is that she'll probably outgrow it by four months of age. In the meantime, you can start trying to unravel the mysteries of colic by reading *The Baby Book: Everything You Need to Know About Your Baby from Birth to Age Two* by Sears and Sears (Little Brown, 2013). If you have a high-need baby, read on. We'll tell you how you can make life with your baby not just bearable but downright rewarding.

"If you didn't hold your baby so much, she wouldn't be so clingy," Grandma (or your lemonade-drinking neighbor) may say.

Or maybe you've said it yourself to your baby's mother. Some people think that high-need babies are made, not born. These people wrongly assume that if you hold a baby too much, the baby will learn to expect, and demand, constant attention. They think that if you give the baby plenty of alone time, she will become easier. Studies show the opposite: The more a baby is held, the more independent she eventually becomes, and the more a baby is left to cry in the first six months, the more she will cry in the second half of her first year. Ask any high-need baby's parent (recognizable by the slightly bouncing walk, the bulging biceps from baby lifting, and the unusually alert baby in a sling) if the little one was born an easy baby. After laughing, a little hysterically, the parent will smile at you, smile at the baby, and say, "Nope, but she's worth it."

High-need babies can easily become much more strongly bonded to whichever parent does the most holding, and this usually ends up being Mom. When Dad comes home from work, he may try to do his share, but the baby seems to think that Mom's hip is softer, and Dad has a difficult time keeping her happy. The logical thing to do is just hand the baby back over to Mom. But a high-need baby who develops a strong preference for Mom will want nothing at all to do with Dad when separation anxiety sets in, between 9 and 15 months. This leaves Mom burned out and Dad left out. It gets worse if Dad agrees with Grandma that Mom is spoiling the baby and so decides to avoid holding the baby to minimize the

The more a baby is held, the more independent she eventually becomes, and the more a baby is left to cry in the first six months, the more she will cry in the second half of her first year.

spoiling. Dad risks missing out on having a close relationship with his child.

If you have a high-need baby, it is critical for you to bond with your baby just as strongly as Mom does, right from the start. This will take a monumental effort. You'll be tempted to hand your baby back to Mom when the fussing starts, because the baby seems to immediately stop crying when you do so. Mom may even grab the crying baby out of your arms, because you just don't seem to be as good with the baby. If your mate does this, have her read this chapter. She needs to give you a chance to be a dad.

We're going to tell you how to become a pro at holding, bouncing, and rocking so your baby will come to cherish your unique touch as much as Mom's. This way, when your baby is six months, one year, and two years old she'll have two parents she's thrilled to be with instead of one she clings to and one who is left out. Pull out that Super Glue, and let's get started.

First, fussy babies love being held like a football. Not the way a center snaps the ball, or the way a quarterback brings the ball up to pass. Try that and your mate will never let you get your hands on the baby again. No, babies prefer the running back, who holds the ball snuggled horizontally against his chest with one arm. We call this the football hold, and there's virtually no baby alive who doesn't love it. Go grab your baby right now (tell her mom you're taking her out to play football), and place her tummy-down along one arm, with your hand in her crotch, her head resting in the crook of your elbow, and her face turned to the side. This position is soothing because the ball of your hand pushes into her tummy. And because the hold is one-handed, you can pat your baby's back or let her suck on your finger for added comfort.

You may find your baby loves to also be swaddled. Being wrapped up warm and tight may remind her of the womb. Swaddling isn't easy, but if your baby is a fusser, you'd better learn to swaddle fast. Here's how: Place an open blanket on the floor with one corner folded down. Place your baby on her back with her head on the folded part. Wrap her right arm in the blanket, bring her right arm across her chest, and tuck the blanket edge under her left side. Bring the bottom corner of the blanket up over your baby's body. Wrap her left arm in the left side of the blanket, fold the arm across her chest, and tuck the left corner of the blanket behind her right side and back. As we said, it isn't easy. But practice makes perfect, and mastering this fine art can really pay off.

Some babies, however, prefer to be loose. Try both to see what your baby likes best.

Fussy babies also love bouncing. Gentle bouncing up and down, from side to side, and back and forth reminds these babies of being in the womb. The more you bounce your baby, the better you will get, and the more useful you will be in your mate's eyes.

Dr. Bob recalls how bouncy he was with his babies:

"One day I was holding our little guy and doing the baby bounce back and forth. I handed him off to Cheryl, and she started the

bounce. A minute later she looked at me like I was an alien (she does that a lot) and said, 'Why are you still bouncing?' I didn't even realize I was. The baby bounce had become automatic."

Rocking is similar to bouncing, except that you do it sitting down. And rocking is one-directional, back and forth, not three-directional like bouncing. So when a baby is really upset, rocking won't be enough. You have to get up and do the bounce for a while to calm her down some, and then you can settle back in to rocking. Mom may give you only two minutes to calm your baby before she steps in, so don't waste time on rocking.

Now we come to sucking. Your pinky may console your baby just as well as Mom's breast, as long as the baby isn't hungry. So have that pinky finger washed and ready when your baby needs it. See chapter 5 for a reminder of the best way to let your baby take your finger.

"Why can't we just use a pacifier?" you ask. You can. But a pacifier feels nothing at all like a breast in a baby's mouth, and a pacifier used in the early weeks can interfere with your baby's learning to take the breast. (Your finger can also interfere, but this is less likely since your finger feels more like Mom's nipple in the baby's mouth. Ask your mate if the baby's latch on the breast feels wrong after she's been sucking your finger. If so, try to minimize the finger sucking for another week or two.) After the first month or two, it's fine to use a pacifier if your baby needs to suck a lot.

A final technique that has proven useful for dads is the neck nestle. Hold your baby upright, chest to chest, with her head snuggled under your chin. Quietly hum or sing as you walk or bounce around. The vibrations from your voice box will be very soothing as they move through your baby. You can also try "shooshing," a mixture of humming and shhhhh-ing. This is what Mom's blood flow through the uterus sounded like to the baby, and it can really take her back to the womb. Also soothing for your baby may be the sounds of a vacuum cleaner, clothes dryer, dishwasher, and hair dryer. Hey, just carry Baby in a sling as you do all the housework, and she should be as happy as can be!

You may find evenings seem to be the toughest. When you are winding down, your baby will be revving up. That's the last thing you need after a long day at work, but if Mom has been home all day with the baby, she'll be drained, too. You are going to have to find the energy to arrive home ready and willing to take over baby duty. If the baby won't even let you both sit down for dinner, stand and bounce while you eat and let Mom have a break and a hot meal. This is your connection time with the baby anyway.

Dr. Jim remembers his daughter's fussy evenings:

"She was fed, changed, warm, and held, but we still couldn't get her to relax. Trying to hold and soothe a fussy baby can try anyone's patience, so Diane and I took shifts bouncing her in the sling. Lucky for us, the fussy stage didn't last long."

A high-need baby is both a challenge and a blessing. For the next few years your baby and toddler will need all the love and attention you can muster. That's the challenge. The blessing is that, if you meet her needs in a sensitive and understanding way, she will blossom into an independent, outgoing, self-confident child. Join your mate in a high-touch style of parenting your high-need baby. You will all be closer for it.

DADA
12

Grandma Can Be Your Best Friend

You and your wife are just beginning to settle in and enjoy the new baby when along comes your mother-in-law to "help." A visiting relative can be a real lifesaver for any new mom and dad. But sometimes the way a grandma chooses to be helpful may interfere with you developing your own parenting skills. And you may have to play referee if your mother-in-law is helping too much in ways your wife doesn't need. If it's your mother who is visiting, there may be even more friction. Let us give you some hints about how to make sure Grandma's visit is pleasant for everyone.

The timing of Grandma's visit is important to consider. You may find you want help right away, especially if you have older children or can't take time off work. But if this is your first baby, you may want to keep your household a threesome while you are home to help. Plan Grandma's visit for when you will be going back to work.

When Grandma arrives, start off on the right foot. Give her a big hug, and tell her how excited you are to be a new dad and how happy you are to have her there to help around the house so you and Mom can concentrate on the baby. She may have thought she was coming to help with the baby, not with the house. She may think you two new parents couldn't possibly be capable of caring for a baby, not until she teaches you how. Since she did such a wonderful job of raising your wife (or raising you), she knows exactly how to raise babies right.

If you and your wife feel the same way, you'll probably welcome all of Grandma's lessons. The only drawback will be that you won't develop your own intuitive parenting skills. You'll be doing everything her way.

Before you learn too much from your mother-in-law, ask your wife how she was raised as a baby and young child. Does she want to be the same kind of mom her mother was, or does she want to do some things differently? She may have a wonderfully close relationship with her mom and want to imitate her in every detail, or she may want to do the opposite. You should also discuss how *you* were raised and what type of mother and father your own parents were.

Assuming that you both feel confident in your ability to learn intuitively how to care for your baby, you may have to prove to

Grandma that you can do this. You—Dad especially—may have to pass the test. You can do this by radiating confidence, by holding your baby throughout the day so you bond with him right from the start, and by showing how good you are at comforting, changing diapers, and dressing and burping the baby. Don't just tell Grandma that you know what you're doing, because she won't believe you. If she sees you sitting on the couch with a beer watching the football game while your wife is walking around the messy house with a screaming baby, Grandma will think to herself, "Boy, do I have my work cut out for me." If instead she sees you walking around the house with a happy or sleeping baby in your arms while your *wife* is resting on the couch in the tidy living room (that you straightened up the day before) sipping lemonade in her bathrobe with freshly washed hair, Grandma will think to herself, "Wow! Now, here's a happy new family. They don't even need me."

You don't want to totally rob your mother or mother-in-law of the joys of being a new grandma. She has probably had visions of sitting in a rocking chair feeding the baby a bottle while you and your mate go out to dinner or catch up on sleep. You want Grandma to feel useful *and* to get used to the baby, because there will come a day when you want to go out for dinner baby-free. It's important for your parents to bond with your baby. Each adult who cares for your child teaches her unique lessons about life and makes her feel more loved. You should encourage this bonding.

A good way to ensure that Grandma's visit begins and ends on a harmonious note is to talk openly at the start about how you

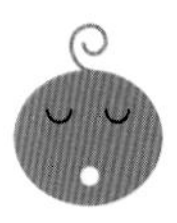

No matter what kind of relationship you have with the grandparents, it's up to you and your wife to control the kind and amount of advice you're getting from them.

and Mom are coping and what you feel Grandma can do to help. If Mom is breastfeeding, tell Grandma that there probably won't be any bottles in the early weeks, but that she can help support Mom's breastfeeding in the same ways you do (see chapter 7). You can also ask her to help you keep the nest tidy so you can spend more time with the baby, but don't expect her to do all the errands and chores for the sake of fatherly bonding. If you do your part, she can have time with the baby, too, and you won't get too dependent on her.

There are several ways Grandma can help you get ahead before she leaves. She can help you shop and stock the pantry. Have her prepare several of her best casseroles to go in the freezer; these will become easy-to-prepare meals for you and your mate weeks after Grandma is gone. Ask her to help you give the house a good cleaning and wash and fold the laundry before she goes home.

In most cases, a visiting mother or mother-in-law is a blessing. But sometimes even the best-intentioned grandparent can undermine new parents' confidence in themselves. You certainly won't do everything exactly the same way either of your mothers did. What will Grandma do when she sees you doing something "wrong"? If she is wise, she will keep quiet and let you learn as you go, unless you ask for help. Some grandparents, however, can't resist making little suggestions about baby care. For new moms especially, these friendly suggestions may seem like veiled criticism. A confident new mother can brush off unwanted advice if she knows Grandma will be leaving soon. But a less confident new mom may begin thinking about every little thing that Grandma says about the way she's raising her baby. She may change her parenting style to fit these suggestions. She may stop trying to meet her baby's unique needs in ways best suited for the baby.

Grandma may say, "Oh, you aren't going to give the baby any formula at all?" or "My, what skinny little legs the baby has." These are perfectly natural comments from someone who breastfed only briefly or not at all. But a new mom may hear, "You can't possibly believe that your milk alone can satisfy your baby. She needs some formula to grow big and chubby." This may cause a mom to doubt her breastfeeding capability. Grandma may also suggest that "babies need to cry sometimes" or "you are going to spoil that baby if you hold her too much." If you and your wife have begun to care for your baby in a responsive, intuitive way, these comments may make you doubt yourselves and change your approach to dealing with the baby's cries. Observe the interactions between your wife and Grandma, especially if Grandma is your mom, and support your wife if you see any conflict arising.

If you are lucky, you and your wife love the way you were raised, enjoy a close relationship with both sets of grandparents, and welcome any bit of advice they throw your way. But no matter what kind of relationship you have with the grandparents, it's up to you and your wife to control the kind and amount of advice you're getting from them. You know your baby best. As long as you trust your own instincts—not rules you learned from a parenting book, but your true instincts—you and your baby will be all right.

13

You Can Keep a Wireless Connection to Your Baby from Work

You've spent a week or two at home getting to know your new baby and helping the new mom get settled. Now it's time to go back to work (as if what you've been doing for the past week hasn't been work). You may be glad that you'll be getting out of the house to enjoy some peace and quiet at the office. Or maybe your job is very stressful, and you've been dreading the return. Whatever your situation, that baby with whom you've spent every waking hour will now be separated from you for eight to twelve hours every day.

You're probably starting to feel the heartache already. We know we did, every day that we had to go back to work. But take this feeling as a good sign. No pain, no gain, right?

So, how can you stay connected with your baby and mate in your triple role as breadwinner, father, and husband? Here are some ideas.

If you haven't started back to work yet, consider taking an extended family leave. Not only would this give you more time to help Mom settle in with the new baby, but it would allow you more hands-on bonding time as well. Establishing a firmer connection with your baby from the start creates a closer permanent bond by allowing more time for the Super Glue to dry. An extended leave may not be financially feasible, but give this option some serious thought before you jump back into your job. The Family and Medical Leave Act may give you a legal right to stay at home longer without any consequences to your career.

Once you do go back to work, run home for lunch, if you live close, so you can get a nice dose of baby. Hold your baby in one arm while you eat with the other. Mom can hang out with you or do some things for herself while both her hands are free.

If your job permits, you might sometimes have Mom and the baby join you at work for lunch. Letting your boss and superiors see you with the baby may buy you some sympathy and a little slack for a few weeks. Ask your mate to drop by your workplace not only for lunch but whenever errands bring her your way.

Even during his pediatric residency, Dr. Bob managed to stay close to his family:

"I had to spend every fourth night working in the hospital. We lived nearby, so my wife would bring the kids over for a quick family dinner in the cafeteria. That really helped me stay connected, and after being at home with the kids all day, Cheryl really craved the adult company for dinner."

Technology can help you stay in touch, too. You might set up a webcam at home and another at the office so you can get an occasional glimpse of the baby and hear his little voice during your workday. As he gets a little older, he'll start to notice you, too. Seeing your face and hearing your familiar voice will help your baby feel connected to you. Mom may be able to send you a digital picture or two every day so you don't feel too out of the loop. Once your baby becomes vocal, a quick phone "conversation" is also nice. And if you are one of those really sensitive dads, a recording of baby's cooing and gooing is fun to listen to halfway through the afternoon (just don't let anyone at work catch you listening to it).

Most men take their jobs very seriously, as well we should. But now you have an even more serious commitment to consider. You are a dad. Your baby needs time with you, and you need time with your baby. We like the anonymous quote on a poster on our office wall: "A hundred years from now, it will not matter what my bank account was, the sort of house I lived in, or the kind of car I drove, but the world may be different because I was important in the life of a child."

Working twelve-hour days five or six days a week doesn't lend itself well to being an involved father. We know that some dads must work long hours to make ends meet for their families, and we commend this hard work and commitment. Some of these dads have the energy and drive to be involved fathers despite such work hours. But if you are working extra-long hours just to make your Ferrari payment and keep up your country-club dues, you may want to take a fresh look at your priorities. Financial success should allow you *more* time off work, not have you so obsessed with your career that your new baby loses out on you.

If your financial situation allows, see if you can arrange to work half-days once or twice a week. This can greatly reduce the shock you may be feeling now that you are away from your baby for a large part of the day. If your job requires you to travel a lot, see if you can temporarily change roles at work so you can stay in town for the next several months. You may not make that promotion you were bucking for as quickly, but in your family's eyes you'll be CEO for a lifetime.

Away from work, try to find ways to incorporate the baby into your activities. If you exercise (and you *should*, as we'll discuss in chapter 25), include the baby in your routine. We often see moms pushing babies in jogging strollers; why shouldn't dads? If you have a home gym, set the baby in a swing or infant seat so you can see each other and "talk" during your workout. If your baby is a morning person, a morning walk with the baby in a sling could be a refreshing way to enjoy a little bonding time. Mom would probably love the extra sleep, too.

Keep in mind that your baby isn't the only one who's missing you. We know that your mate has loved having you at home for a week or two, and now that she has a baby to care for, she'll probably miss you more than ever. If she can't get out much with friends or coworkers, she is probably craving adult interaction. Send her a text or two from work each day, or keep in touch over the phone. Make up for your time away by reconnecting during the evenings and weekends (we'll tell you how in chapter 23).

Try not to let too many chores eat up your home time. Take inventory of all the things you do around the house every week. For example, do you spend four hours every Saturday mowing the lawn and doing the gardening, or washing and polishing the cars? You may have always enjoyed these physical routines, or perhaps you are looking for an excuse to get out of them. Either way, realize that your time at home has become more valuable. Consider hiring a gardener to keep up the lawn or a neighborhood kid to wash the cars. Delegate whatever time-consuming tasks you can so you can make the most of your time at home. Also, try to set aside any hobbies or other distractions for a couple of months so you can focus on your family each evening and weekend.

You will soon find that there isn't enough time in the day to be a full-time worker, full-time dad, and full-time husband as well, just as Mom is finding that the same is true for her roles. How do you balance it all? We have no idea. We still don't have it all figured out. But we manage to do a pretty good job of balancing our marriages, careers, and fatherhood in a way that makes each role fulfilling for all involved.

DADA
14

You Have to Help Keep the Nest Clean

You've had a hard day at work. Traffic was a nightmare, as usual. You look forward to coming home to a nice clean house, being greeted at the door with a kiss from your wife, sipping a cocktail while you put up your feet (possibly to be massaged by your adoring wife), and then enjoying the nice meal your wife has lovingly prepared (since she has had nothing to do all day except take care of one easy little baby). That's your fantasy.

Now let's switch to the new mother's reality. She's slaving away at home all day figuring out your newborn, trying to keep the house somewhat tidy, wondering when she'll get five minutes to grab a quick shower, and counting the minutes until you can come home to give her a break. The last thing on her mind is how sore your feet are. As for dinner, hey, you can microwave your own TV dinner, buddy.

Now, maybe you have a Stepford wife who magically manages to keep a clean house, serve a five-course dinner, and keep your baby well fed and nurtured. But we real-life husbands have to pitch in and help with the chores if we want things to be at all as they were before Baby. Truthfully, your life never will be the same as it used to be. Instead of insisting that your house and life run as smoothly and easily as in the old days, change your mind-set: Life is now, and always will be, different.

So you don't know how to run the vacuum cleaner, and you have no idea how to separate the laundry into lights, darks, and delicates. Or maybe you do. Surveys show that men share in the housework more today than they did 20 years ago.

But there are a lot of things besides laundry that you can do to help keep the house neat. After all, when Mom is stumbling around in the dark at night with your baby—and you're taking your turn as well, right?—you don't want either of you to trip over something.

Besides, don't you think your mate shares the same feelings about the chaos around her? She probably wishes she could do everything around the house that she used to. She may even be worried that she's letting you down. After all, you've been cut off

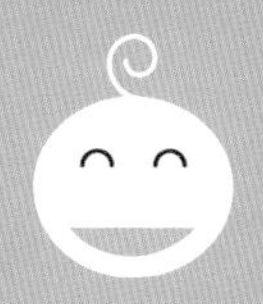

Surveys show that men share in the housework more today than they did 20 years ago.

from sex for six weeks. The least she could do is tidy up a bit and cook something now and then, right? She may be worried you are thinking this way. Or she may be taking full advantage of her new get-out-of-housework-and-cooking card. Maybe she's thinking, "Yeah! Now all I have to do all day is take care of a baby! No cooking. No cleaning. No sex. I have the easy life!" We can almost guarantee you she has no such thoughts.

Dr. Bob learned to be useful when he became a father:

"I can't stand a messy house. Honestly, when baby number one came along, I was a little irritated that the house was messy. Exactly what was my wife doing all day anyway? Couldn't she find a few minutes to pick up? But then she began to describe just how tough her days were, and I realized that, if we were to live in a clean house, more of the cleaning would have to be done by me."

How about you? Do you expect your wife to do it all? We hope not, because by taking care of your baby she is doing it all. Her cooking and cleaning will return later, when the baby is a bit more predictable. For the first month or two, life is all about the baby. So instead of spiraling down into squalor, here are a few things you can do to help keep the nest tidy.

If you have the money, hire a cleaning service to do the dirty work once a week. Be sure to tell your mate you're not doing this because you think she can't handle the work. Tell her you would just rather she focus her time on your baby and herself. This also gives you more time to be with her and the baby. Companies and individuals who offer general postpartum help can be useful, but we suggest you don't let them take over the baby care. It makes no sense to hire someone to hold and feed the baby so your wife can mop the floor. Hired help should let the new mom be a mom.

Find out what your mate likes to do around the house and what she doesn't. If you've been together for a while, you may have determined this already, as Dr. Bob did:

"Early on in our marriage I discovered that my wife hated emptying the clean dishwasher (her daily chore when she was a child), but she loved washing the dirty dishes. So cleaning out the dishwasher became my job, and I almost never had to do the dirty dishes."

Talk together about each of the daily chores that need to be done around your house. You may find that your preferred cleaning duties complement one another very well. And when they don't, flip a coin. (Offer to do the coin toss, and pretend your wife wins every time.)

Next, take notice of some smaller jobs around the house that don't seem to get done regularly. Make a list of these, and tape it to the kitchen cabinet. Tell your mate you've done this as your own reminder, lest she conclude you've put up a list of chores you expect *her* to do. As you walk past this list every day, take note of what needs doing. These should be really quick tasks, things you can do in just a few minutes: changing the cat litter, giving the kitchen floor a quick sweep, or getting the mail out of the mailbox. You can't assume, of course, that the things you choose to do are at the top of Mom's need-to-be-done list. You might ask your partner to name three things that should go on your list to do every day that will dramatically raise the level of her happiness. Dr. Bob was surprised at his wife's request:

"One of the things my wife loved was for me to empty the garbage frequently instead of letting it pile up, stuffing it down with my foot, and taking it out once a week. But I had no idea that she wanted me to empty the garbage more often until we talked about how I could help."

Dr. Jim remembers life before Baby:

"Since there were no kids in the house, Diane had plenty of energy left over to do almost all the housework. She enjoyed keeping a tidy house and rarely asked me to pitch in. I kept myself busy doing much of the outdoor work. When Baby arrived, Diane still would have liked to do the housework herself, but since so much of her energy and time were spent with the baby, I soon realized that the cleaning wouldn't get done unless I did it. And unless I did it, I would have to deal with a tired, worn-out, emotional mom who was also irritated because her house wasn't clean!

"When I first 'inherited' the task of cleaning the kitchen after dinner, I figured this was a temporary arrangement, just until the babies were out of infancy. Well, almost 12 years later, I still find myself doing the dishes while Mom is upstairs getting the kids ready for bed. There was nothing temporary about this shift in responsibilities. I have become accustomed to turning on the TV to watch whatever baseball, football, or hockey game happens to be on while I clean the kitchen. Later, when Diane comes down-

stairs and sees a nice and tidy kitchen, I score major points—*and* I've watched the game!"

Another way you can help is to call home when you're leaving work every day and ask your mate if she needs anything from the store. Stopping to shop will delay your much-anticipated cocktail and foot rub, but going to the store lugging the baby along is a major task for a new mom (try it yourself and you'll see). Your mate will love being able to rely on you to grab that missing ingredient essential to the night's dinner—hey, she's making dinner!—even if it is just hamburger meat to go with the Hamburger Helper.

Perhaps one of the ways you can be most helpful is to pick up five things every night before bed. These will probably be your own things anyway (shoes left in the hallway, jacket thrown over the chair, and so on).

Of all Dr. Bob's efforts to help around the house, he has a favorite:

"Every now and then, when Cheryl had had a busy evening with the baby, I would pull the waking-up-to-a-clean-kitchen trick. I'd throw everything into the dishwasher and run it as she nursed the baby to sleep."

But, remember, being a new dad and a good husband isn't just about helping around the house. Sure, these efforts are appreciat-ed, but what a new mom really loves is having a partner who is an involved father and a caring and sensitive husband. Don't neglect these roles; they are most important in the long run. For now, don't just whine that your house is all a-clutter. Be part of the solution.

DADA
15

You Can Have a Rewarding Career as Mr. Mom

For the most part we have assumed that you are a new father working outside the home to support your stay-at-home mate and new baby. But this isn't necessarily so. Maybe your spouse will also be returning to work soon, or perhaps she already has. Maybe *both* of you are caring for the baby while running a business out of your house. Perhaps you are both working separate shifts and you're taking the day shift at home while Mom takes nights. Or maybe you've simply chosen to be a stay-at-home dad while the mother of your baby returns to a career outside the home.

You may have heard some negative comments from family members and friends about your being a "Mr. Mom." Judging from our experience in talking with stay-at-home dads, such stereotypes are simply not valid. Most men don't choose to stay at home because their wives could make more money or are more career-oriented. And most career moms with at-home husbands don't "wear the pants" in the family. These dads most often decide to stay home mainly because they want to. In our practice, even the dads with "tough-man" jobs are taking a few turns per week as Mr. Mom. With jobs as pilots, firefighters, or police officers, many of these dads have daytimes free. They watch the baby while Mom goes off to her part-time job.

A job's main function is to support a family, and perhaps Mom's job better fits the bill at this time. Mom's job may provide better medical insurance and other benefits for your young family. Maybe Dad's work would require travel, but Mom's doesn't. Or Mom's job may be more stable in the current economy. So, instead of both parents working, the two of you decide to have Dad take the more important job—staying home with the baby. Whatever decision is best for your family is a decision to be proud of.

If you have chosen to be a stay-at-home dad, we applaud you. We've never yet met a full-time dad who regretted his choice. And don't worry that your baby will be getting the short end of the stick. An at-home dad can be just as nurturing as an at-home mom. In this chapter we will share some ideas on how you can make the most of your time at home and how you can help your mate stay connected with the baby.

If you're not a stay-at-home dad, some days at work you probably wish you could be. In any case, please don't skip this chapter. It's not about how to feed and burp a baby all day. It will give you some useful insight into how the other half lives (that's *your* other half, if you have a stay-at-home wife). Unless you've been a stay-at-home parent, you can never really appreciate how much work it actually is. We would like you to do a little role-playing. Pick a Saturday that Mom can spend at a spa or on a long outing with a friend. Make sure you have plenty of milk to feed your baby. Then be a stay-at-home dad for an entire day. This will give you a greater appreciation for what Mom goes through while you are at work. Dr. Bob recalls:

"Even during my years as a pediatric resident, I had the feeling that my wife worked much harder at home than I ever did at the hospital. This feeling was reinforced whenever I found myself in charge of the kids all day. By the end of the day, I was more exhausted than after even the most grueling days at the hospital."

A full-time stay-at-home dad has an extra responsibility—helping Mom stay connected to the baby. Although it can be tough for a dad to leave his new baby all day, it is usually even harder for a mom. You can make the separation somewhat easier on her by following some of our tips in chapter 13, such as setting up a webcam, sending texts and digital photos, and keeping in touch by phone.

But there is much more involved in helping a working mom stay connected to a baby, especially if she is breastfeeding.

You've already read about how important breast milk is for a baby. If Mom has committed herself to pumping at work and continuing to breastfeed at home, you must do everything you can to support her efforts. You should both be familiar with how to pump and store breast milk and prepare and feed with bottles. These details are beyond the scope of this book, so we refer you to *The Baby Book: Everything You Need to Know About Your Baby from Birth to Age Two* by Sears and Sears (Little Brown, 2013). In a nutshell, though, this is what is involved: Mom pumps in the weeks before returning to work to build up a reserve of her liquid gold. When she returns to work, she pumps with a double-sided electric pump at least every three hours to maintain a good milk supply. By law most large employers must provide a private room, not a bathroom, for pumping. We suggest you use the milk she pumps each day to feed Baby the next day so you don't have to freeze it. You can even bring Baby to work over the lunch hour so Mom can feed and connect with him. It is critical that you don't minimize the importance of Mom's milk. Praise her daily for what she is doing.

If your wife is struggling with pumping and maintaining a full milk supply and is thinking of calling it quits, you can get help from La Leche League (877-452-5324) or a lactation consultant (see chapter 7). This can be invaluable in helping a mom.

Working moms seem to never get any time off. They work all day, then come home and work all evening, night, and weekend as mothers. If your mate overextends herself, she'll probably get burned out.

During the night, Mom will need to nurse the baby at least once or twice to maintain her milk supply. This will be much easier for her to manage if the baby sleeps in your room. Even if Mom isn't breast-feeding, she'll stay better connected to the baby if the baby sleeps close by, either in your bed or in a bedside bassinet. If you and your mate were hoping to get the bed to yourselves so you could get back to, well, mating, consider how valuable this extra time will be for both Mom and your baby.

When your baby wakes crying during the night, who gets up? Since you can't use the "I have to go to work tomorrow" excuse, you will have to share in night duties. But if Mom is breastfeeding, it's important for her to do so at night to keep up her milk supply. In this case, avoid bottles during the night. But when it comes to nighttime diaper changes, burping, and soothing, it's important that you do your share.

Even though your wife will be at work all day, she will still be a full-time mother. This means that she's going to spend much of the day wondering what you and your baby are doing, worrying that everything is all right, and hoping that the baby is eating enough, napping well, crying very little, and getting plenty of stimulation from you. When she comes home she'll probably spend the evening soaking up all the baby she can get. She's not going to kick off her shoes, grab a beer and the remote, and recline in her favorite chair to watch the six o'clock news. Working moms seem to never get any time off. They work all day, then come home and work all evening, night, and weekend as mothers. If your mate overextends herself, she'll probably get burned out. So don't think you get to go off duty every day at six when Mom comes home. You'll still need to do your share in the evenings. Perhaps the best approach to evenings is to let your wife take care of the baby while you attend to dinner and other household routines. This gives you a break from baby duty and lets Mom and the baby reconnect.

So, what will you be doing with the baby all day, anyway? You'll do much more than care for the baby's bodily needs as described in chapter 8. You'll find that feeding and changing diapers takes up only about half the day. It's also your responsibility to nurture the baby so she develops mentally, emotionally, and physically. This doesn't mean just setting aside an hour a day to play with her. If you "wear" her in a sling, you can give her the stimulation she needs while doing other things around the house.

Caring for a baby gives you an excuse to take life slower. Take a daily walk with your baby. Hang out in the park. Do errands on foot instead of driving. These are simple pleasures most modern men miss out on.

Focus on your baby when she's awake. When she naps you can do things that require concentration, such as paying bills, studying (if you are a student), or working (if you have a home-based business)—or enjoy a well-deserved break to watch *Star Trek* or play video games uninterrupted.

When the baby is awake, beware of the TV trap. It's all too easy to set a baby in front of a video for an hour to keep her entertained. Just because the videos are named for famous scientists or composers doesn't mean that your baby will grow up to be a genius if she watches them all day. Research has shown the opposite to be true. Babies and toddlers who watch excessive TV are more likely to have learning disabilities, attention deficits, and behavioral problems when they start school. The American Academy of Pediatrics recommends that babies watch no TV in the first two years. This also means that *you* shouldn't watch the TV all day, even if it's sports or news, or the baby will spend too much time watching as well.

No book can really tell you exactly how to be a dad all day. You will learn as you go. Just give your baby all the love and interaction you can to help her grow and thrive into a happy child, and help your mate be the attached mother she wants, and needs, to be.

DADA
16

Dual Careers Are a Dual Challenge

Your baby is almost six weeks old. You remember there was something significant about that six-week mark. Hmmm, what was it? You know it was something important, something critical, something you were looking forward to. Oh, yeah. Sex! You get to have sex. Well, that's a different chapter. There's something else that may happen at six weeks, and it doesn't involve sex. Six weeks may be when Mom's maternity leave runs out. For many American families, this is the time when a new mom returns to work outside the home. You may already have returned to work and learned to adjust to being away from your baby. But Mom hasn't.

And, believe us, she hasn't been anticipating that six-week date as eagerly as you have. She's probably been dreading it. Hopefully she's prepared herself mentally for the inevitable change and is determined to make the best of it.

We've shared some ideas about how to adjust when you go back to work, and we've discussed how to help your wife adjust if she is going back to work and you're staying home. But now it's both of you. You are both going to come home after a long day, take off your shoes, sit back on the couch, and expect the other person to bring you a drink and rub your sore feet. Sure, you could do this for each other, except for one thing—the baby. Maybe one of you could hold the baby while the other person does the foot rubbing, and then you could switch.

It's not that easy. Since the two of you will be sharing the traditional roles of primary breadwinner and primary caregiver, your daily life with a new baby will be far from traditional. Balancing dual careers with parenting will take all your energy. You can do it, and you can each build as close an attachment to your baby as you would as stay-at-home parents. But we won't lie to you: You'll have to work harder at it. Here are some ways you can stay close to your baby and to your mate, remain healthy despite the stress, and enjoy your new role as a father, all at the same time.

If neither you nor Mom has gone back to work yet, take a careful look at your finances and think about the following alternatives to dual full-time jobs. First, one of you might work part-time. Can't decide who gets to stay home more? Flip a coin. But if Mom is

Since the two of you will be sharing the traditional roles of primary breadwinner and primary caregiver, your daily life with a new baby will be far from traditional. Balancing dual careers with parenting will take all your energy. You can do it, and you can each build as close an attachment to your baby as you would as stay-at-home parents.

breastfeeding, she automatically wins. You could also try to arrange extended family leave for one or both of you. Even better, take family leave one at a time. Perhaps you could start back to work first while Mom takes her leave, and then you could take a month or two off when Mom goes back to work. Many large companies have generous family-leave policies, and more laws are being passed to protect a new parent's right to stay home for a period of time. One of you could also consider starting a home business instead of resuming your current job. After Dr. Bob's wife quit her job to stay home with their first child, she provided a home daycare service for two other babies. This was a lot more work than taking care of just her own baby, but the money allowed her to stay home with him. The sooner you start planning, the more likely you'll be able to take advantage of any of these alternatives.

For the hours you will both be away, you must choose the right daytime caregiver. This is tough. Perhaps the best choice is Grandma, if she is available. What better person than the woman who gave birth to you or your mate? If Grandma lives nearby, she may be able to come to your house to watch your baby there. This avoids driving time for you. And Grandma may do it for free. If she doesn't live nearby, you may want to consider having her move in. We know this probably isn't your first choice, or your third, but the advantages for you and the baby may outweigh the inconveniences.

If Grandma is out touring the world, has a full-time career, or just says no, a nanny who comes to your house is the next best thing. Of course, a nanny costs more than group daycare, and you may find that you would have to spend a large part of one of your salaries to pay for her.

If hiring a nanny isn't feasible, a family daycare home is the way to go. Choose one close to Mom's workplace, if possible, so she can go over on her lunch hour to get some baby time. If you can't find a good daycare home near Mom's workplace, look for one close to your workplace. If family daycare stretches your budget too far, consider a workplace daycare center, if either your employer or Mom's provides one. Workplace daycare is generally the least expensive child-care option, and being able to see the baby a few times during the day is a great bonus.

The last choice to consider is a large daycare center unassociated with your place of business. Although a daycare center may be less expensive than a family daycare home, you may find that the drawbacks—less personal care, more driving for you, and possibly, no way to see your baby during the day—outweigh the cost savings. Plus, you'll generally see fewer runny noses at a small daycare home.

Once you and your partner are both back at work, you may find early mornings to be especially stressful times. Following are some ways your family can stay more connected during your busy morning routine.

If your jobs are in the same part of town, drive together to work, and drop the baby off together along the way. This way your baby gets to see both of you each morning, and you spend some extra time with your spouse as well. Driving together also allows one of you to sit in the back seat with the baby in case he's a car-seat

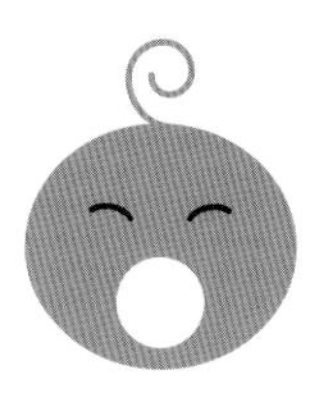

screamer (some babies hate car rides).

If your workplaces are distant from each another, take turns driving your baby to daycare. Then you will both feel involved in your baby's morning. If Mom is breastfeeding, though, it may be better if she does the drop-off and pickup on most days. Nursing the baby upon arrival at daycare may save her one daily pumping.

Try giving your baby an early bedtime so he'll be an early riser. Although having your baby awake makes it more difficult to get ready for work, most babies are happiest first thing in the morning. Letting your baby hang out with you while you shave, dress, and eat breakfast may start the day off better for all of you.

Then again, you may find you like keeping the baby up late for more evening time together. Evenings, however, tend to be fussier times for a baby, and in the morning you may end up having to leave before the baby wakes. He may prefer to wake up to his two favorite people every morning.

In the preceding chapter we shared ideas about supporting the working mother in her breastfeeding and pumping routine. The same advice applies if you are both working outside the home. But with the added stresses of two careers, it is harder to coordinate Mom's milk supply and make sure the pumped milk goes with the baby each day to daycare. Since Mom is doing all the pumping, consider stepping up to be the milk manager.

In whatever form it takes, your support will help prolong the breastfeeding relationship. And continued breastfeeding helps prevent infant illnesses. This means a happier baby when you are

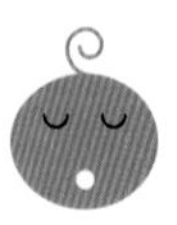

Babies spend a lot of time in light sleep. This means they can sense who and what is around them while they sleep. Your baby will know you are there at night and feel much more connected to you.

together after work and on weekends, and less time off work to care for a sick baby (although, if you think about it, a sick baby gives one of you a perfect excuse to stay home with the baby for a few days).

When you and your mate are both working, one of the most critical ways to stay connected with your baby is to let him sleep with you. If your baby sleeps in another room, he may see his mom and dad for only an hour or two each morning and a few hours in the evening. This is about 20 percent of your baby's day. At the same time, he is spending about 40 percent of his time in daycare. Spending the eight hours of overnight time with your baby really helps. If you are a deep sleeper, you may not notice the baby in your bed very much. But babies spend a lot of time in light sleep. This means they can sense who and what is around them while they sleep. Your baby will know you are there at night and feel much more connected to you. And sleeping together makes it easier for the breastfeeding mom to give the baby one or two night feedings, which are essential for maintaining her milk supply.

If both you and your partner are spending eight hours each day at work, two hours driving, five hours taking care of your baby, and eight hours sleeping, you are left with only one hour for yourselves. You have little time for exercise, and most of your meals are fast food or takeout because you don't have time to cook. This busy routine not only puts a strain on your relationship but also puts stress on your bodies and taxes your immune systems. This may not be a problem over the short term, but after a few years of a high-stress lifestyle, your health will begin to suffer if you don't take good care of yourself.

How can you both stay healthy through it all? A consistent exercise routine and healthy eating habits are key. Not only do these keep your body in shape, they boost your mood and energy levels. Pick an exercise activity that you can all three do together, such as jogging or walking every evening around the neighborhood. Or buy two home exercise machines that you can use simultaneously while the baby watches. If simultaneous exercising does not work, try to develop a routine you can follow on your own during your lunch hour. Ride your bike to work every day, if this is practical. Then you can watch the baby while Mom exercises in the evenings.

Instead of spending the entire weekend cooking, cleaning, and catching up on household duties, try to enjoy some family time outdoors. This helps relax you and renew your spirit for the coming week. Also, pay attention to what you are eating. Both Dad and Mom can apply the nutritional ideas in chapter 25.

Think you don't have enough time for exercise or healthy eating? Without these you and your mate are likely to end up more exhausted at the end of each day, with very little energy left to enjoy your baby, much less each other. You'll spend your little free time sitting on the couch sulking about how tired you are and how little time you have for each other. Years of this downward spiral are unhealthy for any family. If instead you spend active time together and support each other's healthy eating habits, you'll have more energy for yourselves and your baby, get sick less often, and even have more sex (cool!).

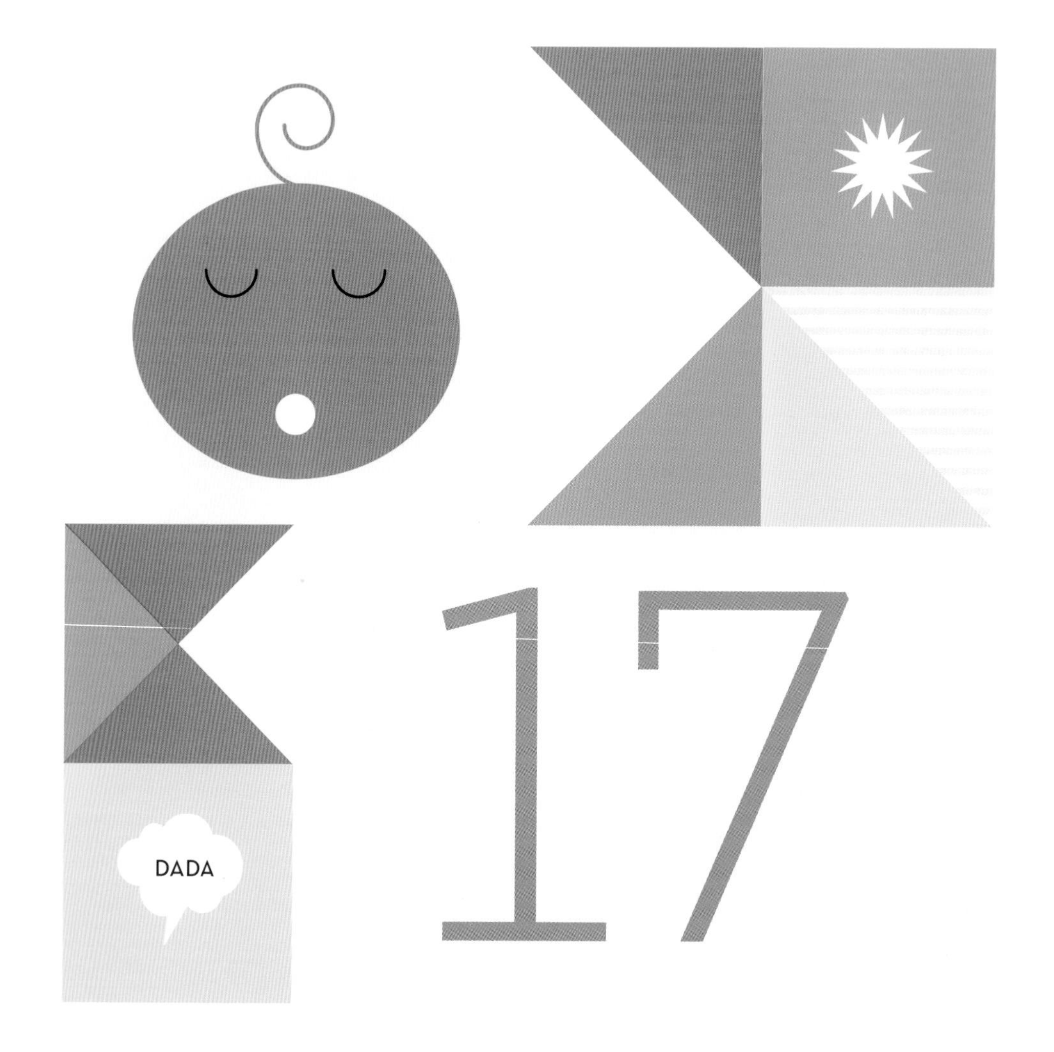
DADA
17

You Can Have All the Free Time You Want

For a new dad, perhaps one of the most devastating things to come along with the first baby is the complete loss of time to oneself. At least Dr. Bob found it devastating:

"I am naturally an introvert. I thrive on alone time. This is not to say I don't enjoy some company. I'm as sociable as the next guy, when I'm forced to be. Before kids, my evenings with Cheryl went something like this: We'd get home from work (which for me was medical school), enjoy dinner together, catch up on each other's day, watch some TV or a movie together, or perhaps play a game or two, or maybe go out for some fun or go to bed early (but not to sleep). And somewhere in the midst of all this I would grab about a half hour to read, watch *Star Trek*, read, study, watch some sports, or read. I always needed that bit of 'me time.'

"When the baby came along, not much changed, actually. We did all the stuff we used to do; we just did it with the baby right alongside. But there was one thing that changed, and that change was BIG. Things would settle down in the evening, and I'd sit down on the couch with a sigh. As soon as I would open a book, I'd hear, 'Honey, can you bring me a diaper and new outfit for the baby? He leaked again.' No problem, right? One minute later I'd be back with my book. Again Cheryl would speak: 'Honey, I'm nursing the baby, and I'm really thirsty. Can you bring me some water?' Easily enough done. Ah, now for my book. 'Sweetie, Baby's done eating. Can you burp him while I start the laundry?' Well, of course.

"Soon I'd have to hold the baby while Cheryl cooked dinner. Then she'd have to take a shower, because the baby hadn't let her in the morning. Then I'd have to change a diaper or two. It soon became obvious that 'me time' each evening was not possible. Or was it?

"Instead of whining about everything the baby, and his new mother, needed from me, I embraced my duties. But exactly how was I supposed to ever be able to read again, much less catch up on *Star Trek*, if Cheryl kept needing my help? It was then that I recognized a pattern in everything my wife asked me to do. Every request she made was either preceded with, or followed by, "I'm _____ing the baby.' Aha! Well, two could play this game. So whenever I sat down to do something all for myself, I just made sure I had that little baby snuggled in my arm. Of course, this left out any two-handed activities, but let me see . . . reading? One-handed. Holding the remote while watching *Star Trek*? One-handed. Studying a textbook? One-handed, with the book propped on my leg. Time alone to myself? Priceless.

"'Honey? Can you clear the dishes off the table while I change the bed sheets?'

"'Oh, no, sorry, dear, I can't. I'm holding the baby,' I'd say, as *Star Trek* played quietly in the background.

"'Darling? Can you empty the trash?'

"'Sure, Love, but later. Right now I'm holding the baby' (and reading my book). I found I could get all the alone time I wanted. And when I got used to wearing the baby in a sling, it got even easier. I'm sure my wife didn't mind, because if I was holding the baby, she wasn't. And it was easiest of all to hold him for his naps. Not only did he nap longer (to my wife's delight) but I wouldn't have to bounce and sway back and forth to keep him content. One of my favorite pictures is of me sitting with my legs up on the desk, sleeping baby in one arm and medical textbook balanced on my legs."

Dr. Jim found his own way of getting free time:

"When my second child was between three and five months old, he was having a hard time getting his late afternoon nap. His older sister, who was about four years old, kept disturbing him. Diane couldn't keep her quiet and him sleeping. I got into the habit of putting him in the car seat and going for a short drive. He would quickly drift off to sleep as we drove over to a local park. I would

arrive in the quiet parking lot, shut off the engine (with the fan still running for ambient noise), and relax with a book for an hour or so. Everybody won: Baby got his nap, Mom got a break, and I got some 'me time.'"

So, how about you? You may not even care about alone time, especially if you're an extrovert. But most every guy needs some time to be a guy. You may call it hobby time or project time or sports time. Whatever it was, it's now gone, or at least much harder to come by. How do you get it back without ignoring Mom and the baby?

Include the baby, and you've got all the free time you need. Of course, the baby doesn't always have to be in your arms. You can set her in a baby swing and let her watch what you are doing. Got errands to run? Take the baby along. Got phone calls to make? Hold the baby while she's sleeping. Basketball playoffs are on? Hey, watch the game with your baby. (But don't let her zone out on it—face her away from the TV as much as you can. And tone down sudden outbursts when your team scores. If you startle the baby, Mom will have to come rescue her, and you'll lose points.) Want to go out and play a round of golf for four hours? Sorry. We haven't found a good way to make that happen.

If you're aching for hands-free time to yourself, either stay up late, wake up early, or don't have kids (we guess that choice is out). Dr. Bob says:

"I learned to grab free time in the early morning. Cheryl and the baby always slept in, but I was an early riser. This was bonus alone time, because my wife was not aware of it."

Anytime you sneak into a corner of the house to get time to yourself, your baby's mother is somewhere in the house taking care of the baby and wondering when she is going to get a break. Who do you think deserves to put their feet up more, you or she? Truthfully, you probably both deserve to rest, but realistically, you'll probably have to take turns. Be a gentleman, and let the lady go first.

Sometimes you and your mate will find yourselves at home together with a napping baby. Hey, simultaneous breaks for both of you. So, what's on *your* mind? Sex, probably. What is *she* likely thinking? A nice quiet snuggle on the couch together. Realize that your couple time is just as important as your individual time alone and is just as hard to come by. In chapter 22 we'll tell you how to get more sex. But realize that a new mom may crave quiet conversation with you, her favorite adult, more than anything else (especially if she spends her whole day talking with herself in babyspeak). Don't neglect the quiet together time every relationship needs. When this need is fulfilled, sex will follow. Not in the same minute, but someday soon.

We'll tell you a secret. Although things are tough right now, they will get better—as long as you don't have another baby right away. Babies don't really get easier as they grow, but you learn how to manage your time, and them, a little better. Don't give up on your alone time. You'll find it if you look hard enough.

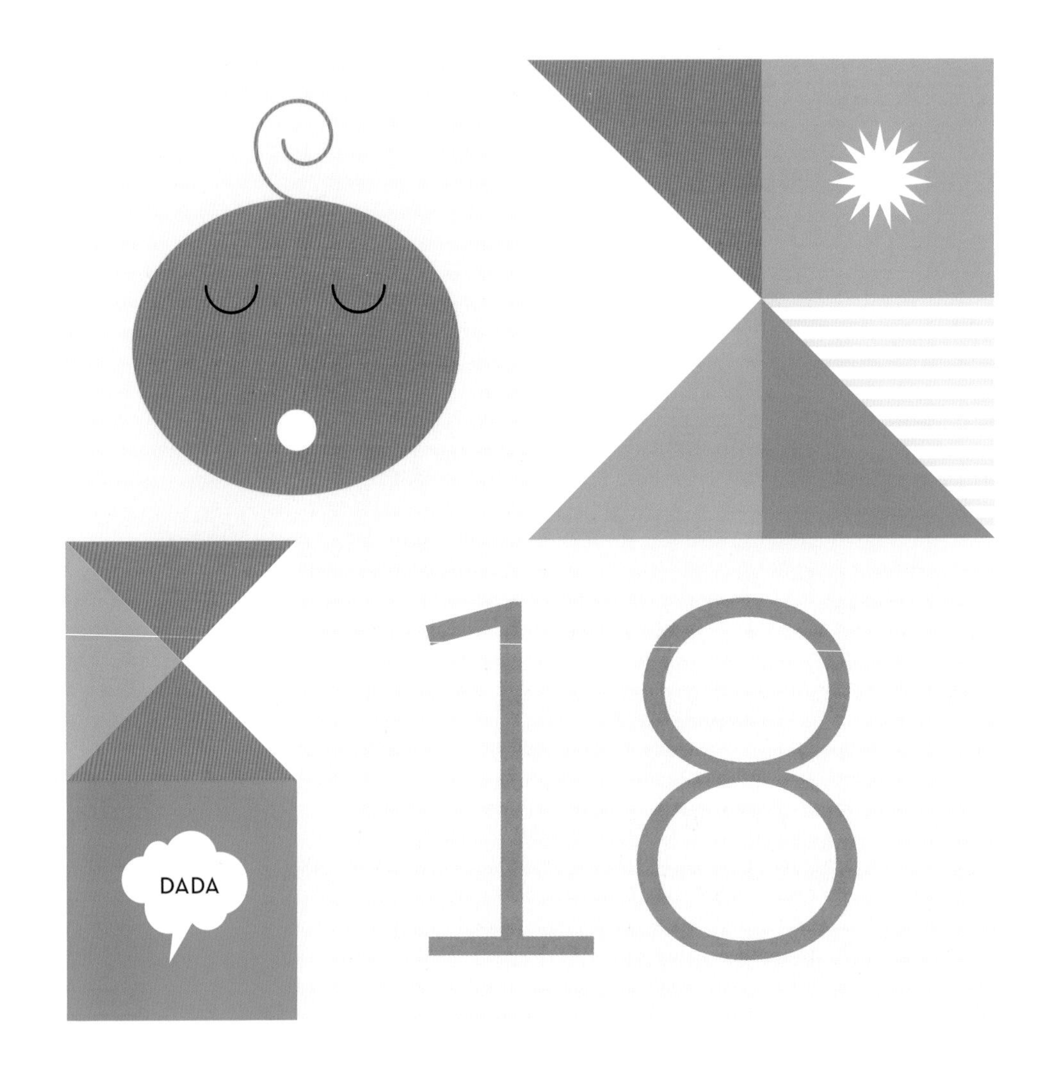
DADA
18

You Have a New Playmate

It will seem at first that all your baby does is eat, poop, cry, sleep, eat, and poop. There's not much for you to do, is there? You don't really need to help with the sleeping, because the baby just *does* that. As for eating, Mom takes care of most of it, if she's breastfeeding. You can help with the crying, but hopefully the baby doesn't do too much of that. So, what else is there?

You'll see as your baby gets older that there will always be more to do than you have time for. But what about right now, in the first months? Does the baby need anything special besides food, diapers, holding, and sleep?

Yes. He needs stimulation. Here's why: A baby's brain starts out very disorganized. The nerves aren't all connected yet. As the baby grows, so do these nerves. As the nerves in the brain and body form the necessary connections, the baby is able to learn new skills. Does this happen automatically? Yes and no. A baby will develop to some extent no matter what you do. He will learn to vocalize, interact, visualize, roll over, sit, crawl, and stand in the first year of life. But to maximize the formation of nerve pathways in your baby's brain, he needs considerable stimulation. The more you stimulate your baby's brain, the more nerve connections will form, and the smarter, faster, and more coordinated he will become.

We'll give you an example: When a baby is born, he can see clearly for about 12 inches. This is the distance from his face to yours as you hold him in your arms. Every second of visual input stimulates the light receptors in his eyes to multiply and form more connections to the optic nerve. This in turn sends impulses into the part of the baby's brain that receives visual input. The nerves in the brain's visual center translate the input into a picture. Every impulse the brain gets stimulates these nerves to grow bigger and longer and to connect themselves to other nerves. This nerve growth occurs in all parts of the brain from all forms of sensory input throughout the first few years of life. If a baby is deprived of vision, the nerves in the vision center will shrink away and die. If a baby is deprived of emotional and social stimulation, the part of the brain that controls emotions and behavior will degrade. This is true for many sections of a baby's brain.

Let us try to put this into manly language. Think of a baby's brain as one big home entertainment theater system (the type of system that was common when our kids were young). A brand-new system gets delivered to two homes. One dad sets up the 52-inch flat-screen TV with a rabbit-ear antenna and a VCR connected by a single cord into the back of the TV. He and his mate enjoy watching TV, when they can get clear reception, and the occasional videotape (when they can't) over the next 18 years without upgrading the system at all. The system is like the brain of a neglected, understimulated baby. The brain functions, but it won't thrive.

Let's meet family number two. Dad sets everything up the same way, but he quickly realizes how poor the reception is. He subscribes to cable to give his system much better input. Then he plugs in a DVD player with not one but four cords and an S-video cable. A couple of weeks later he upgrades to digital cable and buys a DVR receiver. Not satisfied just yet, he runs everything through a stereo receiver so he can watch *Star Wars* through the new surround-sound speakers he just wired through the ceiling. He makes sure that every plug in his system has a cable attached, that

The research results are clear: The more face-to-face interaction a baby gets, the smarter and more outgoing he becomes.

the whole thing is interconnected, and that it is all controlled by one universal remote.

However silly it sounds, this is exactly what happens with a baby's brain for the first three years of life. The more sensory input it receives, the more nerve connections are generated to take full advantage of the information. The result? A happier, smarter, more outgoing baby who turns into a thriving, intelligent, and energetic child.

So far we've been speaking in generalities. Now we're going to talk specifics. What exactly can you do as a dad to maximize the wiring in your baby's brain? Despite our illustration, the answer is not to let him watch TV and soak it all in (although he can listen to all the music he wants). Here are some daddy things you can do to enhance your baby's intellectual, social, and motor development in the first few months:

Give him as much face time as you possibly can. Whenever he is awake and in your arms—about 12 inches from your face, naturally—talk to him, smile at him, and exaggerate your facial expressions. Over the first few weeks he will begin to study your face intently and form facial expressions of his own. You may not get an actual smile for a month or two, but your baby's brain will be soaking in everything you do. In fact, research on children of depressed parents who don't smile, coo, giggle, and do everything else a goofy parent does when holding and feeding a baby shows that these babies have slower social development. And don't worry about overstimulating your baby. The research results are clear: The more face-to-face interaction a baby gets, the smarter and more outgoing he becomes.

Black-and-white contrast is the most stimulating input a baby's eyes can get. Whenever your baby is awake but not in someone's arms, place near him a picture board or toy with black and white stripes or contrasting shapes. He will develop better vision if you do this. Because Dr. Jim's first child loved to watch the ceiling fan slowly rotate, one day he cut some shapes out of dark paper and taped them to the white fan blades. This doubled her enjoyment.

Incorporate your voice into everything you do with your baby. Of course he can't understand your words yet, but you'll love how much more interactive your baby becomes. Hum a tune or have a chat with Baby while you change a diaper, or quietly sing a lullaby while you walk him to sleep.

Other noises can be stimulating for your baby, too. Dr. Jim heard his first baby's first laugh when he quickly zi-i-i-i-ipped open a duffel bag. She would howl with laughter whenever he did this.

What about motor stimulation? You may not care if your baby learns to sing; you may want him to grow up strong and athletic. Well, the best way to stimulate a baby's strength is to hold him upright in your arms. This allows him to exercise his head, back, and abdominal muscles; work on his balance; and practice his hand-eye coordination all at once as he looks around, grabs your clothing and face, straightens his body, pushes against you with his legs, and interacts with you visually through it all. Research has shown that babies who spend more time in their parents' arms develop faster than those who get more floor time.

"But Mom is doing all that," you may say. "Why do I need to do it, too?" If your baby gets all her stimulation from Mom, who is she going to turn to six months from now? As doctors, we evaluate babies' development every day. When we see a baby falling a little behind, we prescribe more touch time from the parents. If Mom seems too burned out to provide more than she already is, we call Dad and give him a pep talk on infant stimulation. But don't wait for your baby's doctor to order you to be a more involved father. Get in there and be a stimulating dad now.

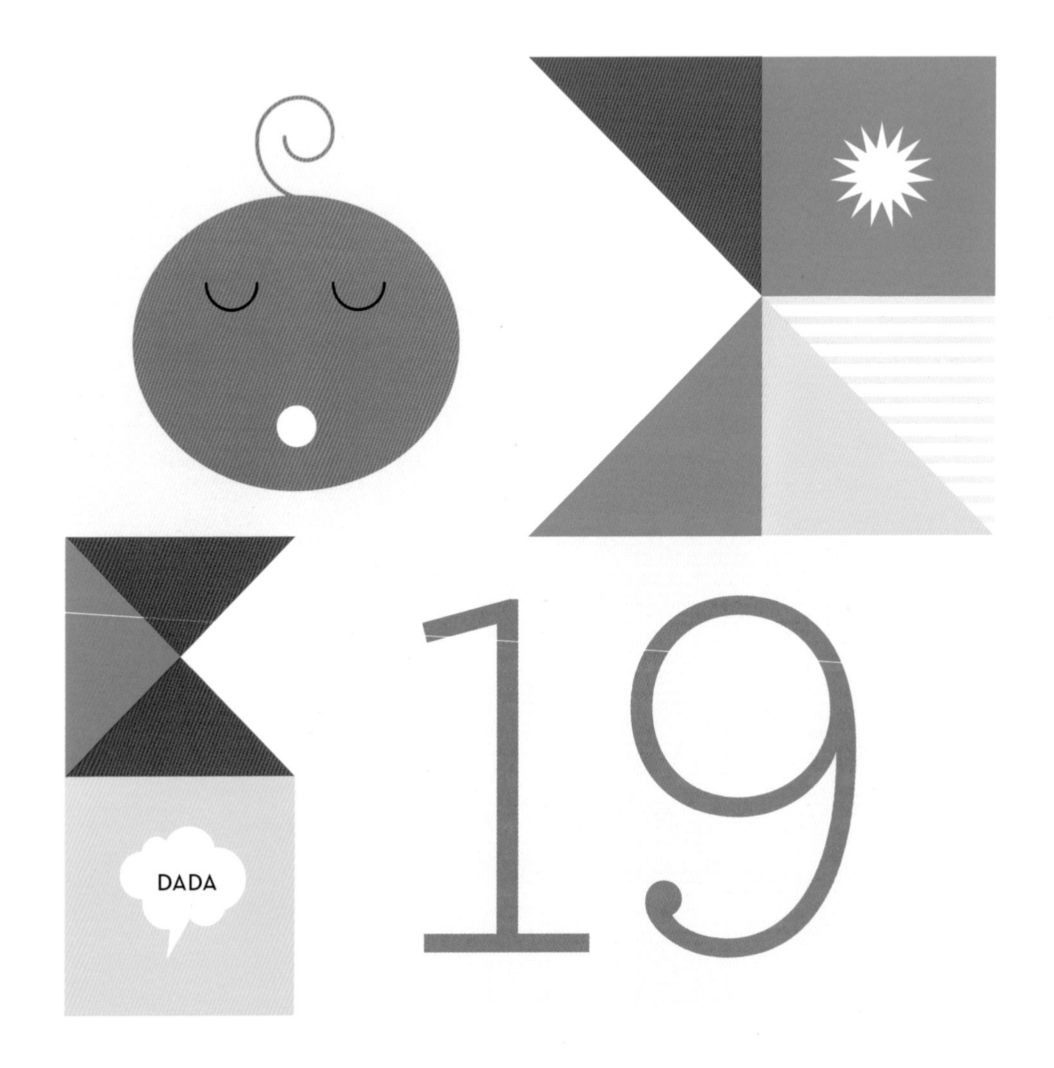
DADA
19

You Can Help Mom Beat Postpartum Depression

The first weeks after her baby's birth should be the most joyful time of a woman's life, right? Well, they aren't always. You observed how pregnancy toyed with your mate's emotions. One minute she was happy; the next she was crying. Now that the baby is out of her, the hormones should return to normal, right? Alas, this is not to be. And we wouldn't want it so, for hormones are the reason she can make milk and develop a mother's intuition.

For most women, the mothering hormone, prolactin, will overpower all other hormonal influences, including that tiny trickle of testosterone (the sex drive hormone) that is floating around, yet well hidden within. Prolactin usually brings out the happy mother. But some women, through no fault of their own, experience an imbalance in the brain hormones that control mood. The result? Postpartum depression.

Normal "baby blues" are a common occurrence among new moms. In fact, 85 percent of women experience some crying, irritability, and anxiety during the weeks after giving birth. Usually these symptoms resolve as Mom's hormones stabilize and prolactin kicks in. But not always.

This is where you come in. It's important for dads to recognize when the normal baby blues have turned into postpartum depression. The difference is in *when* symptoms occur, and for how long. Baby blues are usually gone by the end of the second week after birth. So if Mom hasn't reverted to her normal happy self by that time, or if she becomes depressed a month or two after the baby is born, you should suspect something may be wrong.

Besides depressed mood, particular symptoms to watch for are agitation, fatigue, lack of interest in normally enjoyable activities, poor concentration, difficulty in making decisions, lack of appetite, insomnia, feelings of failure as a mother, guilt, and unusual worry over the baby's health. Any of these may describe your mate at one time or another in the early weeks, but if you notice that she shows four or more of these symptoms much of the day, every day, then you should take action. Be especially watchful if your wife ever had psychiatric problems prior to pregnancy, because if she did, she is very likely to suffer from postpartum depression.

It may be difficult for you to admit that there may be a problem with the mother of your child. No man wants to acknowledge that his spouse isn't up to the task of motherhood. If you find your friends and relatives are expressing worry about your mate, but the possibility of depression hasn't even occurred to you, take their concern seriously.

So, what should you do if you think that your wife is depressed? Sit down with Mom, and share your concerns. You will have to do this in a very sensitive way, of course; an understanding, supportive mate is one of the best treatments for a depressed mom. Try to get Mom to talk about what she is experiencing and feeling.

Call her obstetrician or midwife, and make an appointment for both of you. Usually a postpartum checkup isn't until six weeks after birth, but this is too long to wait if you suspect a problem. The doctor or midwife can refer Mom to a postpartum depression support group in which she can learn to understand and cope with her feelings. A family therapist or psychologist can be invaluable for in-depth counseling. The O.B. or a psychiatrist may prescribe an antidepressant medication for a short time to help get Mom through (most such medications are safe to use while breastfeeding). This should be a last resort, however. There are many things you can do as a family to support a new mom without turning to drugs right away.

Take extra time off work so you can help care for your baby. Your mate will need you now more than ever. So will your baby. If postpartum depression is severe or prolonged, the lack of an emotional connection between mother and baby can have a detrimental effect on the baby's social and intellectual development. You will want to provide the emotional and physical stimulation your baby requires until Mom is able to do so.

Fortunately, studies have shown that breastfeeding protects an infant from the psychological effects of a mother's depression. In other words, the stimulation a baby gets during breastfeeding can be enough to ensure normal development. Research has also shown that breastfeeding women get over postpartum depression more quickly. For these reasons, it is important to encourage Mom to continue breastfeeding.

Breastfeeding difficulties, however, can increase both stress and depression. Nipple pain, a common cause for early weaning, has been shown to increase postpartum depression. It is important to get help for a mom who is having difficulty breastfeeding, and to encourage her to stick with it.

Gather the support of family and friends. But you must make sure that everyone involved is sensitive and understanding; there's nothing worse for a depressed new mom than a condescending mother-in-law to rub it in. If no family members or friends can

The best exercise for a depressed mom is a brisk walk every morning for an hour or two. This helps clear her mind of worry and gives her a fresh start each day.

come to your house to help, consider hiring a postpartum doula to help with the baby and the house every day for a few weeks. At your baby's checkup, tell the doctor about the depression.

If Mom is willing, have her start a simple daily exercise program (ask the obstetrician what is safe, or check a pregnancy book). Exercise, even just two to three times per week, has been proven to have an antidepressive effect. Mom's routine can't be very vigorous in the first several weeks after birth.

The best exercise for a depressed mom is a brisk walk every morning for an hour or two. This helps clear her mind of worry and gives her a fresh start each day. You can either arrange a caregiver for the baby (or you can watch Baby if your work schedule allows) or have Mom take the little one along in a stroller. A family walk around the neighborhood each evening will also lift her spirits. If you live where winter is too cold, invest in a treadmill.

Nutrition plays a big role in combating depression. Many studies have shown that omega-3 oils have the same biochemical effects as antidepressant medications—without the potential side effects. Mom can get plenty of these oils by eating fish several times each week (wild Alaskan salmon is the healthiest). Eggs also have some of these oils. If Mom isn't a fish eater, she can take omega-3 oil capsules (make sure they have DHA and EPA).

Don't tiptoe around your wife all day. Talk about her depression openly with her. Her reactions will help you gauge how she is responding to your interventions. Acceptance of her condition and a willingness to work through it are good signs. Denial and accusations toward you are signs that either you are wrong or the situation is more severe than you thought. Your health care provider, support group, and family can help figure this out.

Having a mate who is struggling with postpartum depression can be a big disappointment. Some dads will express anger over a wife's inability to cope with her new role. The mom, of course, is feeling enough guilt already; she doesn't need her husband to add to it.

You probably envisioned your wife as a perfect mother who would take wonderful care of your baby. She will be that mother someday soon, but you are going to have to take up the slack for a month or two until she works through the depression. If she gets the appropriate treatment, your mate will likely be able to thrive as a new mother and provide for your baby in every way necessary. In the meantime, your extra help at home will give you a much closer connection to your baby.

Although this book is generally lighthearted, there isn't anything funny about postpartum depression—though a dad may smile when he sees Mom break down in tears because the baby's socks don't match the baby's outfit. What we are going to discuss now is even more serious than postpartum depression. We do this with the intent not to worry but to inform you. We refer to something called postpartum psychosis. In this severe form of hormonal imbalance, a woman not only experiences depressive symptoms, but she also suffers symptoms that may include hallucinations, delusions, thoughts of hurting herself or the baby, and severely impaired day-to-day functioning. Postpartum psychosis is rare; it is thought to affect one or two women for every thousand deliveries. If the condition goes unrecognized, though, both the mom's and the baby's lives may be in danger. When this condition occurs, immediate treatment and safeguards are needed.

There is one more postpartum condition you should know about. Studies have shown that some dads go through mild depression after a baby is born. This is due not only to the increase in financial and personal responsibilities but to hormonal influences as well. We urge you to share any feelings of sadness you may have with your wife and your friends. A good exercise routine and healthy eating can also be a great help.

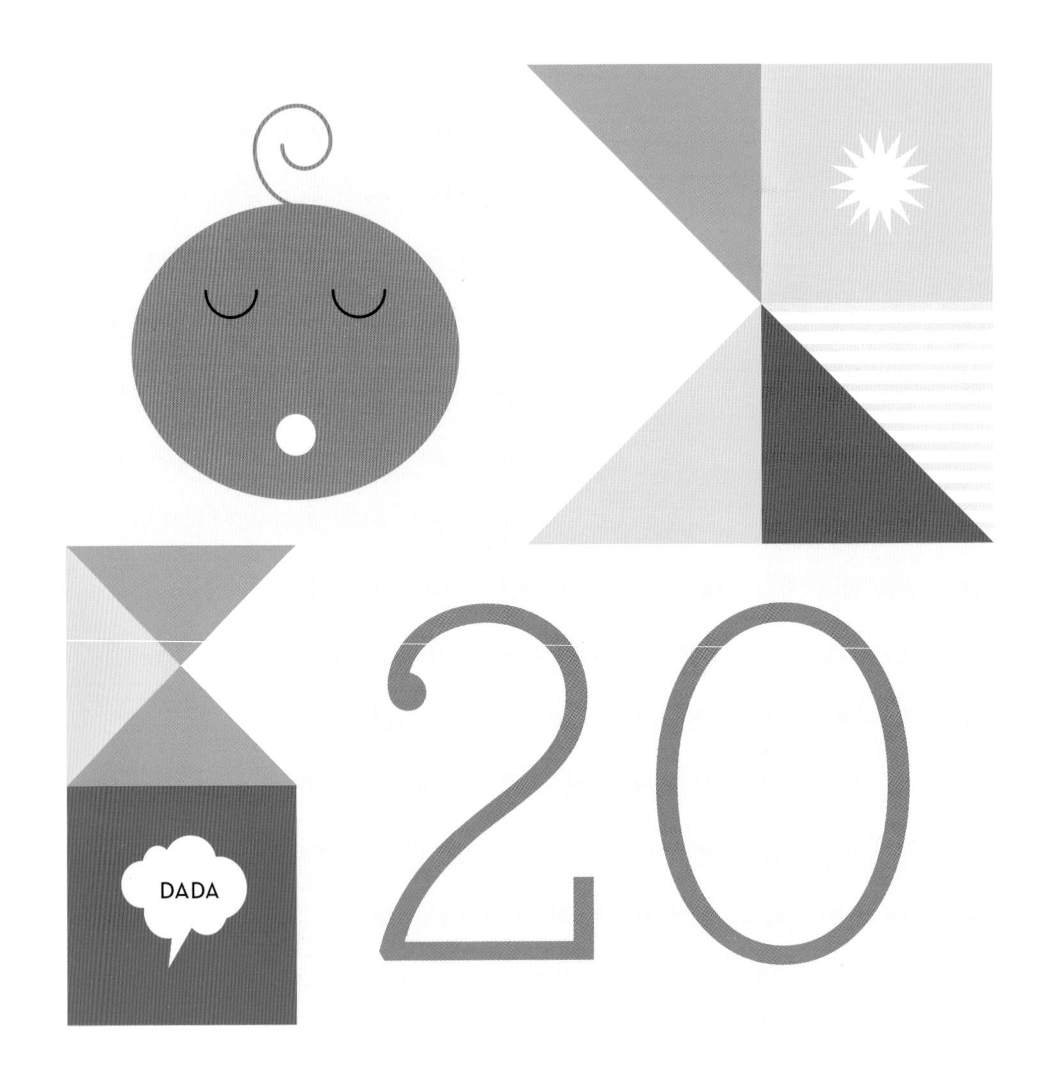
DADA
20

You, Too, Can Sleep Like a Baby

As tired as you must be, we can't believe you're even reading this. One day you were getting eight hours of sleep each night, and then, wham! Not only did your mate keep you up two nights in a row through labor (you did stay awake, didn't you?), but now the baby is keeping you up, too. We often walk into a hospital room to check on a newborn and find the mom sitting up in bed snuggling with the baby while dad is zonked out on a cot in the corner. We whisper to the mom, "Let's let him sleep. He's been through a rough couple of days." As if Mom hasn't!

How do you cope? There must be some way, because dads have been doing it for millennia. Since between the two of us we've made it through five kids, we can throw a few ideas your way to make it a little easier.

A typical newborn sleeps all day and stays up all night. We think this is because he was lulled to sleep as Mom walked around all day while pregnant. When she lay still all night, trying to sleep, the little guy kicked and squirmed inside her. Most parents are thrilled when their newborn sleeps for most of the day of his birth. But then comes the night. It's party time for the baby, and there's really nothing Mom and Dad can do about it.

These first few nights are an initiation into the club. Your baby is testing you to see if you can hack it. Thankfully, he will slowly change over a few weeks into a night sleeper, especially if you wake him often during the day for feedings.

Even if your baby sleeps well at night, he probably still wakes for feedings every few hours. Some dads don't mind this; they happily help with feedings and diaper changes. Our hats are off to you if you cope easily with night wakings. Dr. Bob had a hard first night at home with his first baby:

"It was 10:00 PM and we were all ready for bed (I was especially, as I'd been up for the past two days and nights). We had the cradle next to our bed, the matching baby blanket and sheet, the cute pajamas, and violin music filtering in from somewhere. Cheryl nursed the baby to sleep and laid him gently in the cradle.

We snuggled in bed and fell asleep. Half an hour later the baby woke up crying. Cheryl nursed him again (I had to get up to help her), then put him back in the cradle asleep. Another half hour went by. 'Waaaaaa!'

"'Honey, can you hand me the baby?' my wife asked.

"'What's the cradle doing on my side of the bed anyway?' I thought as I passed the baby over and tried to go back to sleep. A short time later I woke again to 'Waaaaaa!' I guessed Cheryl had fed him and put him back into the cradle while I was sleeping. I grabbed him and handed him over to Cheryl again. 'Why don't you just keep him right there in bed next to you and let me sleep?' That's how supportive a dad I was at two in the morning. But Cheryl listened to me.

"The next thing I knew I was waking up to the sunrise after six hours of uninterrupted sleep. I looked over and saw Cheryl and the baby sleeping peacefully.

"Every night for three years, each of our babies slept right next to us in our bed (one at a time, usually). We didn't plan this; it just happened. And I slept so well almost every night that I'd usually have to ask Cheryl in the morning, 'So how did you and the baby sleep?' She'd either smile, stretch, and give me a pleasant answer, or she'd grumble something unintelligible, pull the covers up over her head, and turn her back to me."

Dr. Jim opted for the guest room whenever he really needed a good night's sleep—such as after a full night on call in the hospital:

If your baby doesn't sleep well by himself but seems to be insisting on sleeping closer to you (well, probably not to you, but to Mom), you may find that the easiest thing to do, at least for the short term, is to let the baby sleep in your bed.

"When the baby wasn't sleeping well, such as when she was teething, my wife would say, 'This might be a night of frequent nursing. You may want to go to the guest room. I'll see you in the morning.' I didn't worry that my baby had replaced me in 'our' bed—I just knew this was the best way to catch up on sleep."

Right now you and your mate are probably in one of two situations. Maybe your baby is sleeping just fine in a crib, a cradle, a bassinet, or your bed. The baby wakes up once or twice each night, you take the wakings in stride, and you really don't have much to complain about. Or your baby isn't a good sleeper and you find yourself getting up at all hours of the night trying to help Mom cope. If your baby doesn't sleep well by himself but seems to be insisting on sleeping closer to you (well, probably not to you, but to Mom), you may find that the easiest thing to do, at least for the short term, is to let the baby sleep in your bed.

You've probably heard that if you let your baby sleep with you you'll never get him out of your bed, he'll ruin your sex life, and you'll be the one who ends up sleeping in another room. Hey, no one ever said parenting was easy. In reality, though, we didn't find any of this to be true. So don't worry about the long term; just try to get a little more sleep. If you let Junior stay in your bed, you may finally get the sleep that's been eluding you.

One way you can have your baby sleep close at hand, but not in your bed, is to get an Arm's Reach® Co-Sleeper®. A three-sided crib that attaches to the edge of the parents' bed, the Co-Sleeper gives

Mom easy access to the baby during the night, but Baby sleeps on a separate mattress so his nighttime squirming won't disturb you as much. You can find this baby bed online.

Now comes the secret to a real full night's sleep. This secret applies only to you; it won't guarantee any more sleep for Mom or Baby. The secret is to encourage Mom to exclusively breastfeed. If you feel so left out of the precious role of feeding your baby that you ask Mom to let you give the baby a bottle, beware. She won't let you give him a bottle only in the evening or on Saturday morning. You're going to feel that elbow in your ribs at 2:00 AM when your baby is crying down the hall. "Go give him a bottle, honey," Mom will say. If you are a selfless superdad who actually enjoys giving your baby a midnight bottle, you deserve a medal. We're sure Mom appreciates your giving her a break. But if you are one of the 99 percent of dads who want at least six hours of uninterrupted sleep, don't ever suggest a bottle, and you'll be off duty at night. If necessary, you can even pull out the Expert card ("The American Academy of Pediatrics recommends exclusive breastfeeding, honey"). Without lactating breasts, you're off the hook.

Now we all know that moms have more stamina, energy, and patience to tend to a baby at night than dads do. But even the best mom in the world needs a break sometimes. Such a night came to pass when Dr. Bob's first baby was about two months old:

"It's still a little fuzzy in my mind, since I was awakened out of my usual deep, uninterrupted sleep. It was around three in the

morning when Cheryl poked me in the rib. 'Here, take your baby. This is his fourth time up!'

"I woke up just enough to catch the baby as he was dropped into my arms. I thought to myself, fourth waking? Is that a lot? I used my powerful dad's intuition to sense that the baby was crying. What did my wife expect me to do? I got out of bed with the baby in my arms (hmmm, so this is what it's like to get up in the middle of the night with a baby—not a very pleasant experience) and walked into the living room.

"A minute later Cheryl felt me climb back into bed. She probably thought to herself, 'How sweet. My loving husband rocked our baby back to sleep, and he's bringing our sleeping baby back into our bed to snuggle with. Ahhh, life is good.' She might have drifted back into peaceful slumber, but something must have been itching at the back of her mind. I think she realized that what she thought had happened was too good to be true. She must have decided to roll over and check to make sure the baby was OK. I was just drifting off to sleep when I heard her very loud and shocked, 'WHERE'S THE BABY?'

"Baby? What baby? 'I don't know,' I mumbled. Why was she asking me where the baby was, anyway? Wasn't it nighttime?

"Cheryl flew out of bed, ran into the living room, picked the baby up off the couch where I had apparently left him crying, and brought him back into our bed. Oh, I thought. That baby. That was the last time Cheryl asked for my help at night with baby

number one, though I got a chance to redeem myself with babies two and three."

Let's be honest. Even the most die-hard mom will sometimes need help at night. We recommend you *don't* follow Dr. Bob's example in this instance. There are many ways you can be supportive, as we'll show you in the next chapter. Be ready to work an occasional night shift. Your mate will love you for it.

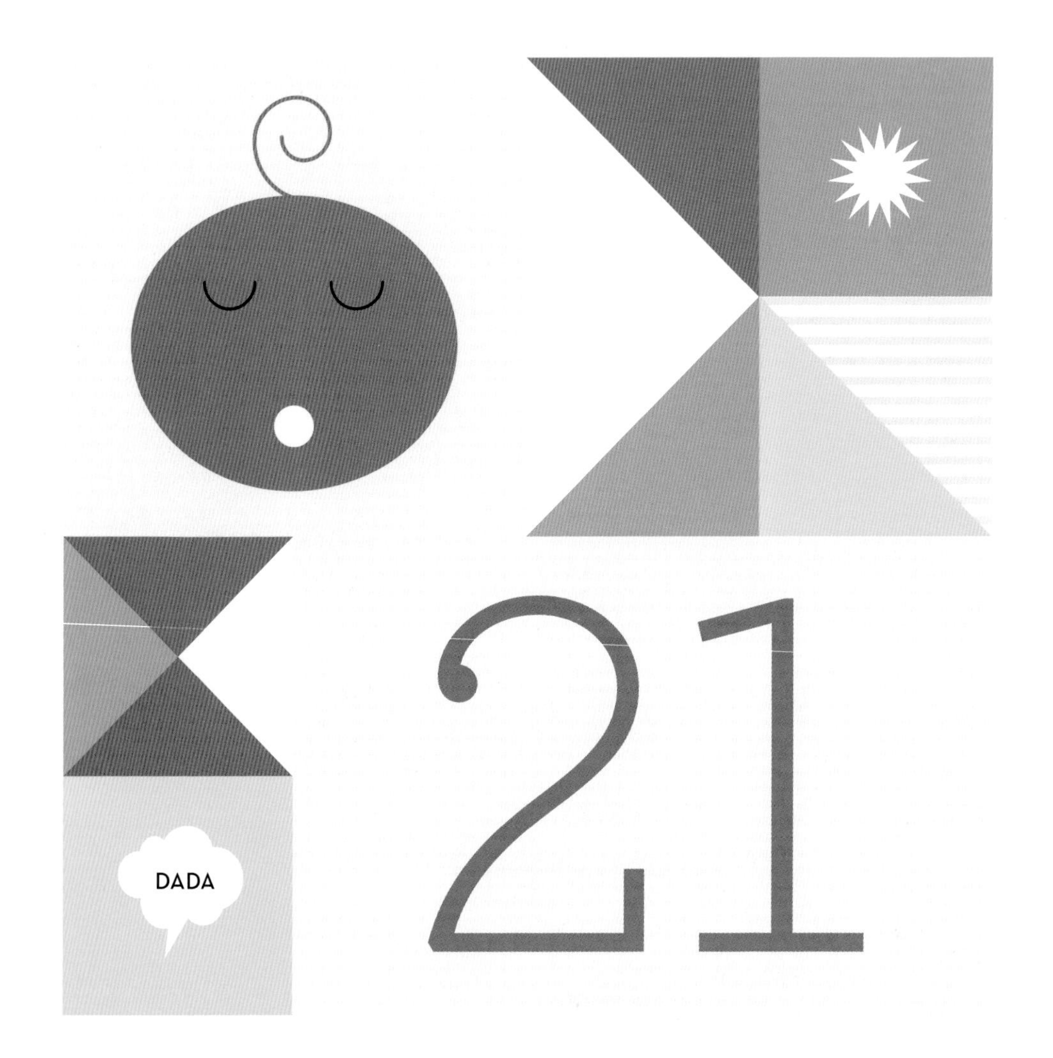
DADA
21

Oh, Yeah—Mom Needs Sleep, Too

Even the most unobservant new dad will take note of the dark circles under his wife's eyes, the way she nods off to sleep while standing in the kitchen preparing his dinner, and the stumbling gait that has replaced the bouncing strides she used to take before the baby came. If you haven't yet noticed these things in the new mother of your child, leave this book for a moment and go check on her. She's probably asleep somewhere in the house (because she was up every two hours last night with *your* baby).

In the preceding chapter we told you how to get enough sleep—for yourself. Now, in case you'd like to stay married, we'll tell you how you can help out at night so your wife can get enough sleep, too.

You are probably thinking, "But I can't help out at night! I have to work during the day!" Men have come to define work as that which causes us to leave the house each morning and return ten hours later with money in our pockets with which to feed our women and children. You want to know what most new moms would call that? A vacation. Go ask your mate right now just how glad she is that you have volunteered to be the worker so that she can stay at home with the new baby and not work all day. She probably won't answer your question with an appreciative hug, a kiss, and a renewal of her vows to you, all in thanks for your hard work that makes it possible for her to enjoy a life of luxury.

In truth, some women find their life with a new baby isn't all that tough. They thrive in their new role as full-time mother, manage to get adequate sleep, and enjoy enough quiet time while Baby naps to do things around the house. Some new dads can return to their careers without needing to be the housekeeper and overnight caregiver. They can come home each evening and just have fun being a new dad. But if your first weeks with the new baby have been more challenging than you expected, take heart. Things will settle down eventually.

Except for the time Dr. Bob abandoned his crying baby in the living room, he doesn't actually remember ever getting up with his babies at night. But Dr. Bob's wife assured him that he did:

"She said there was a second attempt with child number one, when he was about 18 months old. Something about his nursing all night and driving her crazy and her handing him to me and my walking around with him while he cried and his finally falling asleep in my arms and then sleeping through the rest of the night. I have no recollection of this, but apparently my wife appreciated it."

As for our other babies, they were all very good sleepers. But in the first few weeks they woke up a lot, and our wives now tell us that we helped out with a number of nighttime diaper changes and supported their breastfeeding during the newborn weeks. We just don't remember.

Dr. Jim thought his first baby was sleeping through the night at age one:

"I was surprised to learn that the baby was still waking up two or three times a night. My wife would quickly nurse her back to sleep without any fuss. I would sleep right through these awakenings even though they were happening only inches away from my peaceful slumber."

If you're a sleepless dad, this should reassure you: No matter how tough things are at night, in a few years you'll have forgotten all about it and may even consider having another baby.

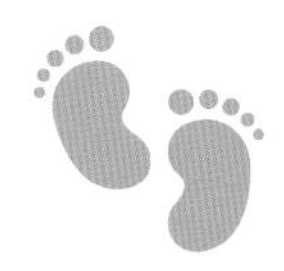

But who are we to say so? We never had a baby who was up every two hours for the first two years of her life. We've had such babies among our patients, but our own babies slept very well right from the start. Sure, they woke up once, twice, or thrice each night to nurse, but our wives were OK with that. This book isn't about *our* wives, though; it's about you and your mate. If your baby is waking a lot and Mom isn't taking well to sleepless motherhood, it's time for you to share the load. Yes, yes, we know you have to be alert and awake for work all day, but what's more important? Your job (at which your coworkers and bosses are likely to ignore your temporary decrease in productivity), or your mate and baby? We hope you answered the latter. In case you want to help out—oh, and keep your relationship together, too—here is advice from the sleepless dads of some of our patients.

Take either the before-bed shift or the sunrise shift (or both, if you're Superdad). If you are a night owl and Mom isn't, then send her to bed at nine o'clock and hold your baby for a couple of hours. When he gets hungry, bring him to bed to nurse, and clock out. If you're bottle-feeding, of course there's no need to wake Mom for this feeding. If your mate is the night person, then let her watch the late show with the baby while you hit the sack early. Then you can get up when he wakes in the morning and enjoy a couple hours of daddy time while Mom sleeps in. (If you're worried about when you're going to have sex on this schedule, see chapter 22.)

When the baby wakes you at night, do whatever you can to minimize the disruption for Mom. Let her stay in bed while you go grab your hungry baby. Help her get the baby settled in for a feeding.

If you're a sleepless dad, this should reassure you: No matter how tough things are at night, in a few years you'll have forgotten all about it and may even consider having another baby.

Change the baby's diaper. Fetch Mom a drink of water. When the feeding is done (if you are still awake), offer to burp the baby and change his diaper (again). Use a dim lamp so Mom can easily go back to sleep while you tend to the baby.

Dr. Jim, a handyman, installed a dimmer switch for the bedroom light.

"This way, we could keep it dark so the baby would stay sleepy, yet we would have enough light to change the diaper. And, of course, I secretly knew the dimmer would be useful later on as 'mood lighting.' (I also tried to convince my wife that our baby would enjoy a mirrored ceiling, but she didn't go for that.)"

Even Dr. Bob assisted with nighttime diaper changes:

"When I heard the baby fussing at night, it usually meant my wife was changing his diaper on the bed beside me. I'd roll over and let him suck on my finger. This kept him calm so he'd fall back asleep more quickly. I'd also make sure my wife had plenty of diaper-changing supplies nearby before going to bed so I wouldn't have to go fetch them during the night. See how thoughtful I was?"

What can you and your mate do to keep yourselves functioning in these early sleep-deprived weeks, besides drink coffee? Lack of sleep will put stress on your immune system and rob you of energy. And if your wife gets sick, *you'll* have to get up with the baby more at night. As we've said before, one of the best ways to boost your immune system and energy level is to exercise (see chapter 25). If you don't have a routine already, start one now. An early-morning walk could do your body good, and it could do Mom good if you bring her and the baby along. Take a multivitamin, eat plenty of fruits and vegetables (or buy a fruit-and-veggie supplement from any health-food store or home distributor) and take some extra vitamin C and echinacea to help avoid catching any colds or flus that come your way.

This night job of yours isn't going to last for long. Most babies wake up several times at night for the first few weeks only. By one or two months of age, most become much better sleepers, and then you are off the hook (at least until teething starts at about five months—then you're back on night duty again). So, be a superdad for the first month. Share in the night duty. Your mate will love you for it.

DADA
22

Sex *Will* Happen Again Someday

No fathering book would be complete without a heart-to-heart talk about sex. Or, more accurately, the lack thereof. This is one of the more difficult adjustments for many new dads. "But we only have to wait six weeks," you may say. "Then we'll be able to have all the sex we want, right?" Dream on. Six weeks is the amount of time doctors say you have to wait to be sure that your wife's body is recovered enough for intercourse. But if you think your wife is counting down the days as eagerly as you are and that on day 42 she's going to attack you and make passionate love to you, you may be in for a surprise. It probably ain't gonna happen.

Why? It's those darn hormones. It seems that female hormones are the excuse for every complaint men have, but in this case they really are responsible, and there's nothing we can do about it.

When a woman gives birth, her brain begins to produce a new hormone, prolactin. Sometimes called "the mothering hormone," prolactin stimulates the breasts to produce milk. It also gives a mom the urge to nurture her baby. Do you wonder why your wife seems to be more immediately responsive to the baby than to you? Why she jumps up and hurries to the baby when he starts to fuss? You can blame it all on prolactin, which surges when a mom hears her baby cry. Prolactin also inhibits a woman's production of testosterone (testosterone creates a woman's sexual drive, just as it does a man's). Prolactin levels remain high as long as a woman is breastfeeding. So although a new mom may be physically ready to have intercourse after six weeks, she may not have the hormonal desire to be sexual for many months.

We dads have a biological disadvantage. Studies have shown that men produce some prolactin after their baby is born, and our testosterone levels go down for several weeks (this is nature's way of giving our wives a break). But we have neither as much biological drive to nurture as our wives (which is why a man should make double the effort to bond with his new baby) nor as much relief from our sexual urges.

Dr. Jim nostalgically remembers the second trimester of pregnancy:

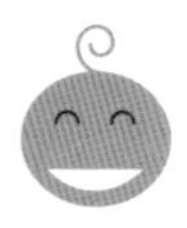

Every woman regains her sexual desire in her own time. It may be within a few months, or it may take a year or two. Blame this on nature, which considers a baby's survival more important than a man's sexual needs.

"My wife's desire for sex increased . . . a lot! Since experiencing these amazing three months, I have spent the past several years trying to re-create this hormonal state in my wife. It hasn't been easy. One thing that has helped is that the kids are growing up and we now have much more time for 'us' without 'them.' I have also noticed that the more energy I spend being a good dad, and good husband, the more my wife is attracted to me, and the more . . . you know."

Every woman regains her sexual desire in her own time. It may be within a few months, or it may take a year or two. Blame this on nature, which considers a baby's survival more important than a man's sexual needs. You can whine and plead all you want (a turn-on for any woman, right?), but in the battle of your testosterone versus her prolactin, you'll lose every time.

There are other reasons a new mom may not feel like having sex. No man can truly understand the amount of physical and emotional energy that a new mom spends on her new baby. By the end of the day (or often by the middle of the day) a mom feels drained. Women have described this as being "all touched out." After feeding and holding a baby all day, a mom may not want anyone else's hands or mouth to come near her. This can be quite a blow to the male ego. Mom's nipples may feel sore in the early weeks. Her lowered estrogen levels may lessen vaginal lubrication. If she had a severe tear or episiotomy during birth, she may fear reinjuring the sensitive area (using a lubricant gel for a few months can make intercourse more comfortable for her).

"She used to quiver when I kissed her. Now she shudders," we've heard dads say. But a new mom does like physical affection that is not sexual. Your mate may enjoy being hugged if she doesn't feel you're coming on to her. She may cherish kisses, but not the kind that linger and increase in intensity. You may groan when you hear a woman in a movie say, "Just hold me!" But now you are in that scene. Your wife will still love your touch, especially at night, but she may mostly want to snuggle. As your testosterone rises, hers may still be hiding somewhere deep in her left toe.

How can you unleash that hidden testosterone? With patience and more patience, understanding, plenty of nonsexual physical affection, support for her mothering role, involvement with the baby, and very patient waiting. The more you share in the baby duties, the more energy your mate will have left for you. If you rock the baby to sleep and get him all tucked in to bed, and Mom finds herself marvelously unencumbered for an hour, who knows what might happen? A relaxing massage from you every night or two also won't hurt.

You might think that after you show such patience and understanding for several weeks your wife will be so appreciative that she'll jump all over you one night as a way of saying thanks. This may happen, but it may not. Your wife may be so focused on the new baby that she doesn't even notice how amazing you are being. Or she may notice and appreciate it, but she may not think of saying thanks with sex. In this situation, some men sulk, pout, ignore their wives, and even resent the new baby.

What can you do instead? Don't expect your mate to read your mind. She may not know that you feel left out, and that you need her to show sexual attraction for you. Sit down with her when the baby is asleep, and tell her how you are feeling (radiate patience and understanding as you do so). Ask *her* how *she's* feeling (women love that!). You may come to a better understanding of each other, which will bring you closer, even if it doesn't lead to more sex right away. At least she'll know what you're going through and you won't have your feelings bottled up inside you.

There's one more thing about sex you need to keep in mind: the potential result! Some women regain their fertility within only a few months, although others may take a year or two. If Mom is exclusively breastfeeding, you can probably count on at least six months of natural birth control, but her menstrual cycle will resume unless she feeds the baby at least twice during the night. Once the baby starts sleeping six to eight hours straight (wouldn't that be nice?), Mom's periods may sneak up on her. And she will be fertile two weeks *before* her period. Some women get pregnant a second time without ever having a period between pregnancies. Until your wife's cycle becomes predictable again, you'll have to take precautions, such as using condoms. Birth-control pills can decrease Mom's milk supply, so we wouldn't recommend them until near the end of the first year.

If the baby is hogging your bed, one question may be nagging at you: Where are you supposed to have sex? Actually, you probably won't even care. You just want sex. When your wife is ready, you can christen every room in the house. Some couples set up a futon or several blankets on the floor in the bedroom to use for lovemaking if their baby is in the way. Other couples are comfortable making love in bed while their baby sleeps in a cradle or other baby bed in the same room. A baby in your bed doesn't have to interfere with your sex life at all.

Every dad experiences a situation that in hindsight seems humorous but at the moment it happens can be very frustrating: You are enjoying your lovemaking when the baby starts crying. You've been waiting all evening for him to go to sleep so you can have your way with his mother, and now the little guy can't even stay quiet for 15 minutes. Do you ask your mate to ignore the cries and stay focused on you? Probably not. We suggest that the first time this happens you let your mate follow her instincts. She may reach over, turn off the monitor, and continue with you. But don't count on it. Remember, her prolactin alarm will start to go off, and even if she wishes she could keep her attention on you, every ounce of her being may drive her to push you away and get to her baby as fast as she can. Talk things through after this first episode. Ask her how she felt when the baby woke up. Decide what you will do when this happens again. If she tells you she must respond to the baby right away when he cries, you'll need to respect this. You may find that as

Baby gets older Mom's prolactin alarms diminish. She may actually demand that you ignore the crying baby for a few minutes while the two of you stay focused on each other. One can only hope.

The good news is that sex will definitely return to normal at some point. Well, almost. There will be that occasional interruption. During this adjustment period, show your wife that you are a mature husband and father. She'll appreciate your patience, and you'll be better for it.

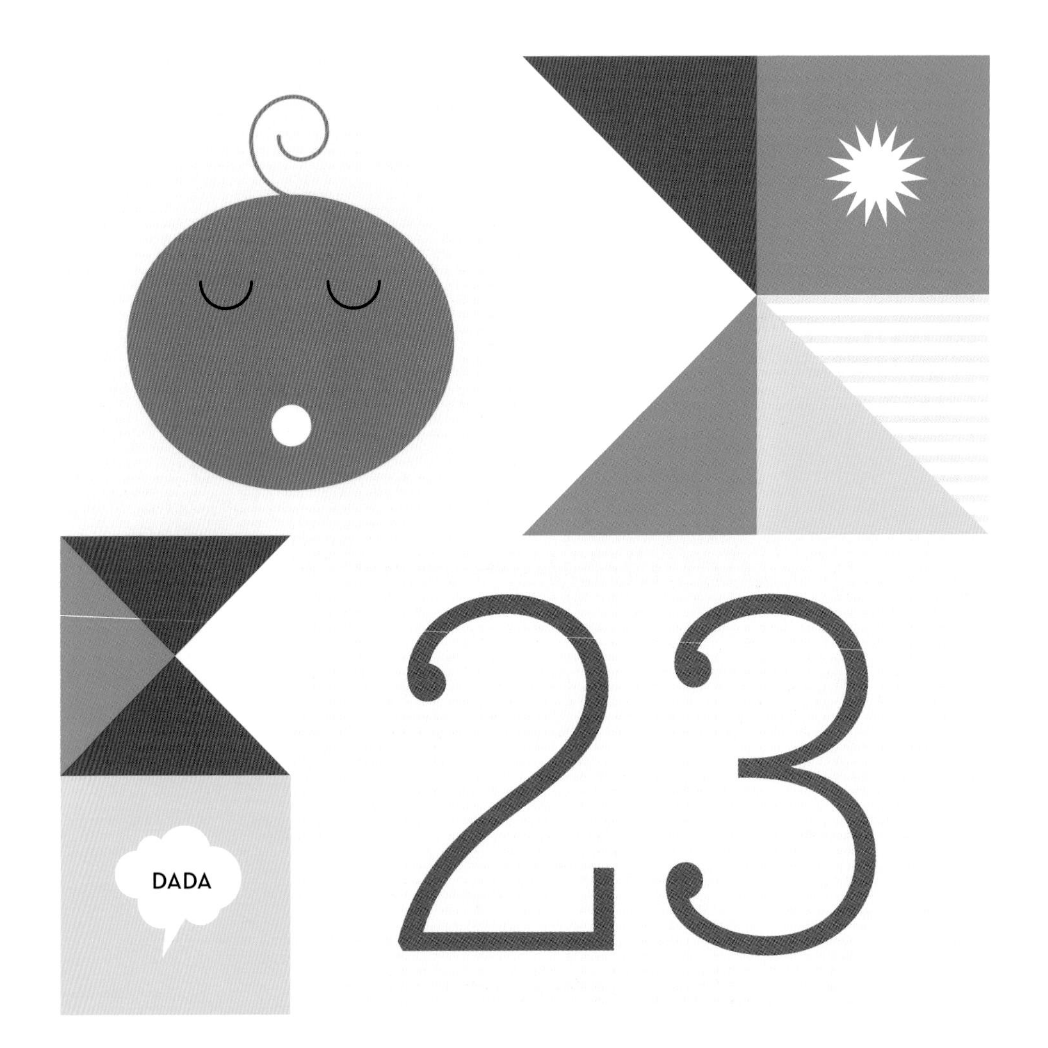
DADA
23

A Good Dad Remembers He's a Husband, Too

Dr. Bob's wife once told him:

"'Bob, you're a fantastic father, and a good husband.' Of course, she didn't say this out of the blue. We were evaluating how our marriage was going. Although I took the compliment about my parenting well, I heard loud and clear the real message behind her words: My skills as a husband could be a little better. I am not just the father of our children; I am also my wife's husband. And I'm not just her husband; I am the husband of my children's mother. I'll give you a minute to think about that. I needed five. . . ."

You can't be a great dad and a bad husband at the same time. When you are raising a child, you are raising someone else's future spouse. If you fail at being a husband, then you may be teaching your child how to someday fail at being a husband or wife as well. Modeling a healthy marriage is a critical part of raising kids. So in reality Dr. Bob wasn't being a fantastic father, and he really couldn't be one until he raised the bar on his role as a husband.

How can you be both a super dad and a super husband? We'll give you a few ideas that we've been thinking about.

First, you and your wife have to make time for each other. Dr. Bob explains:

"I won't say that Cheryl and I focused on parenting too much in the early years, because we wouldn't change a thing about how close we are to our kids. But we sometimes forgot to also put in enough time for each other.

"Now that we have three kids, we are a lot less reluctant to go out on a date. Rather, we look forward to it. We started leaving our third child with a sitter when he was still a baby. But if you'd asked us if we wanted to go out and leave our first baby with a sitter, we'd have stared at you as if you were speaking Latin. Going out without him never even occurred to us. What else was there to do in the evening besides sit at home and play with our baby?

"When I share these comments with the crowd at parenting conferences now, I get blank stares from couples with one child, and nods and smiles of agreement from those with two or more

kids. If Cheryl and I were negligent of each other as first-time parents, maybe we were just doing what comes naturally to most people with their first baby."

Most dads are ready to leave the baby at home long before moms are. Although some moms can't wait to get out without the baby after a couple of months, others don't want to leave her until she is two or three years old. Many moms tell us that they wish their husbands would stop pressuring them to leave the baby with a sitter and go out for a romantic evening just for two. If you manage to get a date alone before your wife is really ready, she'll spend the entire evening wondering how the baby is doing without her while she occasionally remembers to smile, nod, and say uh-huh every few minutes while you talk to her. In this case, you will have to be patient. In the meantime, reserve a table for three for dinner. You probably won't have a candlelight meal with violin music in the background, and you won't be able to go park somewhere and make out, but Mom will appreciate your accepting her motherliness instead of demanding she act like a mate.

Dr. Bob recalls many dates for three with his first baby:

"The baby slept for very long stretches when we carried him in the baby sling. We enjoyed many nice dinners and movies out in the early months while he slept snuggled against us. When he started to wake, Cheryl could easily feed him back to sleep."

If your wife isn't ready to go out (with or without the baby), create a date at home. While Mom puts the baby to sleep, prepare a romantic dinner (cook it yourself or get takeout) with candles and quiet music. You might make this a routine for every Friday or Saturday night.

When your mate wants to start dating again, arranging for a babysitter may still be too much hassle for her. Dr. Bob figured out how to help:

"It seems that Cheryl is always the one calling the sitter, making a dinner reservation, and checking the movie times when we want to go out. So sometimes I take the initiative and make the arrangements myself. Cheryl is always surprised when I call her from work in the afternoon and tell her to make a simple dinner for the kids because she and I are going out.

But sometimes the dad in me can't resist trying to include the kids in one of our dates. I arranged a movie date one night, then said to Cheryl, 'Hey, the movie we're seeing would be fun for our eleven-year-old. Why don't we bring him along, to show him we recognize that he's growing up?' Good idea, right? Not when your wife is home with the kids all day, every day, while you're at work. Cheryl just glared at me. We left our son at home."

No matter how much you value time alone with your mate, you may hate to leave out your baby. Dr. Bob feels the same way:

"Sometimes I feel bad that our third child is missing out on me. He doesn't get every bit of my time as the first did. Neither did our second child. With each child my time is more diluted. But that's an inevitable part of having three kids."

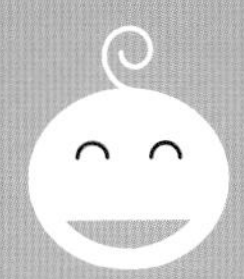

Remember that in the long run your children will appreciate that their parents not only are still together, but love being so.

Remember that in the long run your children will appreciate that their parents not only are still together, but love being so.

As you start your new role as a dad, you may find the romantic side of your marriage gets put on the back burner. You have a choice to make: You can either resent the baby for interfering and resent your wife for her lack of physical attention to you, or you can become the hero of the family. New fatherhood reminds Dr. Jim of one of his favorite movies, *Die Hard* with Bruce Willis:

"It's a story about your average cop who gets thrown into an extremely stressful situation. He has the chance to save the day, to be everybody's hero, and he tackles the situation head-on with incredible bravery and a little bit of luck. When men watch a movie like this they think to themselves, 'Man, it would be cool to be a hero like that!' Well, new fathers, here's your chance to come out of a die-hard situation looking as good as Bruce did. It's stressful. It's hard. You will be tired. But if you tackle the challenge head-on, you will become the most attractive person on the face of this planet in your wife's eyes. This is your chance to rise to the challenge, to be the cream of the crop, to be the hero."

Dr. Bob made an important change in his evening routine as his kids got older:

"In the evenings I used to play with the kids until they went to bed, and afterward hang out with my wife. But then I'd often be too tired to do anything but sit on the couch next to her. Now when I come home from work I first greet her with a kiss (unless

one of the kids greets me at the door), find out how her day went, and then say hi to the kids. I also usually hang out in the kitchen with Cheryl while she's making dinner instead of running around outside with the kids until the third call for dinner."

As your family grows, remember little things like dates, flowers, your time and attention, and whatever else makes your mate feel happy and loved. Take inventory of your marital relationship just as often as you evaluate your role as a dad. Don't neglect one for the sake of the other. And if you think you are going to win the father-of-the-year award, make sure your mate will be there to cheer for you.

DADA
24

You Can Ace Doctoring 101

We see a lot of sick babies in the office. They suffer from everything from rashes to colds to coughs to diarrhea to screaming that the average parent can't figure out. Usually we receive a concise description of the baby's past 48 hours, including temperature readings; the color of the baby's snot; the presence of unusual rashes; the color, texture, and odor of the baby's poop; and an assessment of how bad any cough is. In fact, this accounting of a baby's symptoms is essential to an accurate diagnosis. Our work is usually very easy, as long as Mom is there to help.

But here's what usually happens when Dad brings in a sick baby. We exchange pleasantries with him for the usual 15 seconds before asking, "So what brings you in here with the baby today?" Instead of narrating the history of the baby's problem as just described, Dad fumbles in his pocket to produce a folded, slightly tattered note. "Ah," we say. "It's the note from the mom." Not that we're complaining. We don't expect a dad to pay attention to the subtleties of his baby's illness. All Dad knows is that the baby isn't sleeping, and so Dad isn't sleeping, and it's our job to fix it.

What's worse is when there's no note. Then we end up talking to Mom on Dad's cell phone to get the story.

In this chapter we're going to teach you how to take your baby to the doctor without needing a note. We didn't say without a note (Mom may still want to send along her version of events). We said without *needing* a note. After reading this you'll be able to pay close attention to your baby's symptoms so you can accurately describe them for a doctor.

More importantly, we're going to tell you what you can do to help get your baby through most common illnesses. Here's where you can really shine. When your baby gets sick and Mom seems bewildered, you'll be able to confidently announce, "Don't worry, honey. I know just what to do." Of course she won't believe you at first. You'll have to show her.

The most common illness that babies get in the first weeks actually isn't an illness at all; it just looks like one. Most babies get a stuffy nose that starts in the first week or two and continues until the baby is about six weeks old. The airways in the chest are often congested, too. The baby breathes with gurgles and rattles and sometimes has trouble feeding because he can't breathe through his nose.

The most common illness that babies get in the first weeks actually isn't an illness at all; it just looks like one. Most babies get a stuffy nose that starts in the first week or two and continues until the baby is about six weeks old.

Of course, the first thought that any new parent has is, "Oh, no. My baby has a cold." Mom may want to rush off to the doctor's office, after she's done blaming you for not washing your hands before handling the baby. Hide the car keys. Your baby probably isn't sick. This is just a normal phase that a baby goes through as his sensitive airways get used to inhaling dust, odors, pollens, and everything else we all breathe in every day. The congestion will pass. Calmly reassure your baby's mother that it's just normal newborn stuffiness. When she doesn't believe you, have her read this page.

Now, how can you help the baby? Loosen the mucus by squirting into the baby's nose a few drops of nasal saline solution (buy it from the drugstore or make your own, using ¼ teaspoon salt in 8 ounces warm water) or breast milk (yes, breast milk). Then use a bulb syringe to suction out your baby's nose. Prop him in your arms to sleep, or place a pillow under the mattress so he sleeps at a slight angle. Turn on a steam vaporizer in the bedroom, or hold your baby in the bathroom with the hot shower running. This is usually enough to help him through. If these measures don't help within a week, then see the doctor. Extreme congestion may be a sign that your baby is allergic to something in Mom's diet (such as dairy products) or to the formula you are using.

The next most common newborn illness is, once again, not

really a disease. It's a normal newborn rash. Most babies develop red bumps and pimples on the face, chest, and back, and some get them on the extremities. This is usually nothing to worry about; it goes away by six weeks of age and doesn't require treatment with creams or lotions. The rash shouldn't bother the baby. If he does seem irritated by it or shows other signs of sickness, you can have your doctor take a look just to be sure he is OK.

Here's another non-illness: spitting up. Most vomiting in newborns is just this. Virtually all babies will spit up some of their milk every day, and many will actually seem to bring up an entire feeding once or twice a day. Spitting up isn't anything to worry about as long as your baby generally seems happy and is gaining weight. If your baby is repeatedly fussy throughout the day or night, though, the spitting up may be causing heartburn, indicating possible gastroesophageal reflux disease. Talk to your doctor about this. Also, if your generally happy newborn has projectile vomiting (that is, if the milk shoots out a few feet) more than several times each day with increasing frequency, see your doctor.

Now here's an illness that is a real problem: fever. If your baby has a rectal temperature over 101 degrees in the first six weeks of life, call the doctor right away. Rectal? you ask. Ouch, but yes, this method is more reliable for newborns than any other. You should always have an infant rectal thermometer on hand. Insert it about an inch into the anus, and hold it there for three minutes if it is a regular glass thermometer or until it beeps if it's digital. Don't treat the fever; your doctor will want to see your baby first.

After six weeks of age, you can take the temperature in the baby's underarm and treat a fever with acetaminophen. If the baby then perks up and becomes playful, there is no need to rush in to the doctor. If your feverish baby acts lethargic, that is, he is limp, he won't open his eyes, he won't feed, and he seems as if he's asleep but he isn't really, or cries inconsolably for hours, you should call your doctor right away. These symptoms may indicate an infection that requires prompt treatment.

Babies who have an older sibling or two are likely to catch the common cold. At first you may insist to your baby's mother that this is just the normal newborn stuffiness we've already described. Here is how you can tell if the baby actually has a cold: His nose won't just be stuffy; it will run. At first the mucus will be clear, but then it will thicken and turn white, yellow, and possibly green. The baby will probably begin to cough, too. He'll be a little fussy, and he won't sleep very well. You can then confidently announce to your mate, "Honey, our baby has a cold."

But should you see the doctor for a simple cold? As long as there is no fever, the baby is consolable and able to feed fairly well, and he has no sustained labored breathing in the chest, then you can probably stay home. If the breathing becomes labored (consistently more rapid than usual, with the abdomen or neck caving in with each breath and wheezing sounds like someone makes when having an asthma attack), you should call the doctor right away. Don't worry if the breathing sounds phlegmy, as long as it isn't labored. And don't worry how bad a cough sounds if the baby has no fever and no labored breathing and seems generally happy.

To help the baby through a cold, do what you would for normal newborn stuffiness: Suction his nose and hold him in the bathroom with the hot shower running. At bedtime, prop the baby up to sleep, and use a steam vaporizer in the bedroom.

The last common illness is diarrhea. Nothing causes more confusion than a baby's poop. One day it's yellow, the next it's green. First it's runny, then seedy, then runny again. You can expect your baby's poops to vary to some degree, and as long as he is happy, there's no worry. If the stools become runny or mucousy for more than a week, but Baby isn't really acting sick, this may mean he is allergic to something in Mom's diet or to the infant formula. Your doctor can help you figure this out.

You can tell that your baby actually has a diarrheal intestinal infection when the stools become much runnier, more frequent, and foul smelling. He will also be fussy and may have some vomiting or fever. In this case your main task is to keep Baby hydrated. If Mom is breastfeeding, she should continue as usual. If you are bottle feeding, you can dilute your baby's formula with water or an oral electrolyte solution available over the counter in drugstores, or temporarily change to a soy formula for a couple of weeks (cow's milk formulas are more difficult to digest during a diarrheal illness). There are no medications that will help. If you see blood in the poop or your baby is getting dehydrated (less urine output, dry mouth, and little to no tears when he cries), then see your doctor.

Even if your baby never gets sick, you will still be taking him to the doctor for well-baby checkups. The schedule for checkups varies slightly from doctor to doctor, but in general it goes something like this: The doctor will see your baby in the hospital the day after the birth (if the baby is born at home or in a birthing center without a pediatrician, you'll bring your baby into the doctor's office in the first couple of days after birth). The doctor will probably want you to bring the baby into the office when he's a week old or, if you're formula feeding, when he's two weeks old. The baby's next checkup will probably be at two months (some doctors will do a one-month checkup as well). Then it's four months, six months, nine months, and one year. Now that you know this you can surprise Mom by reminding her to make the appointments. Even better, take an hour off work to go see the doctor with her.

So now you are a medical expert, right? If not, at least you've learned the basics of what to do for common infant illnesses and non-illnesses. Perhaps most important of all, when you take your baby to the doctor you'll be able to describe all of the important symptoms, because you know what to watch for. If Mom slips you a note anyway, read it in the waiting room, and then toss it in the trash. You can handle this yourself.

But don't be offended if we hand you a note with instructions for your baby's mother. It's not that we don't trust you. Well, yes it is. We know that when you get home and Mom says, "Tell me everything the doctor said," she's not going to settle for "Oh, the doctor said everything's fine." She'll want it in writing.

DADA
25

You'll Want to Play with Your Grandchildren Someday

Whoa! Wait a minute—or a few decades. Grandchildren? Who's thinking grandkids right now? Not you, certainly, and neither did we when our first kids were born. When we were just starting our families, thoughts about our long-term health never even occurred to us. We ate all the burgers and fries we wanted. We drank soda as if it were water. Ice cream was our usual midnight snack. And we certainly ate our fair share of the kids' Halloween, Christmas, and Easter candy when they weren't looking.

But now, years later, we take our health very seriously. Why should we even think 25 years into the future? Because we want to be able to toss a football with our grandchildren someday. What we are doing about our health right now will determine how healthy and active we'll be in the future.

What happens to the typical American dad? He has kids, works hard, forgets to exercise, eats an average American diet, and then has a heart attack at age 60. Dr. Bob describes his first health scare:

"I got my cholesterol checked for a life insurance policy at age 30. It came back at 280. My insurance agent called me with the result, asked if I was having any chest pains, and told me to go see a doctor before I died of a heart attack without life insurance. I was shocked. I was an active guy, and I actually had a fairly low-fat diet. I took this seriously, though. By following a very strict diet, I lowered my cholesterol to 180 in two months. And I started thinking: I want to be a healthy, active dad when I'm 55. I don't want to miss my third son's wedding because I'm in the cardiac unit at the hospital. So I stuck with the low-fat diet, started an exercise routine, and tried to limit the junk food. I am determined not only to play football with my kids, but to play it with their kids as well."

Here's the first thing you can do so you can be a dad and a granddad for the next 60 years: Watch your fat intake. The foods people eat often that are high in unhealthy fats and cholesterol are entrées with a lot of cheese; beef; deep-fried breaded foods; ice cream; some crackers, cookies, chips, and other snack foods; and most salad dressings.

Dr. Bob explains how he lowered his cholesterol:

"I read labels on every food I ate. I not only checked for cholesterol; I looked at the grams of fat as well. If anything had more than 15 grams of cholesterol per serving, I did not eat it. If it had more than 10 grams of saturated or trans fats, I did not eat it. I began eating chicken instead of beef. I often ate a large salad (with low-fat dressing) instead of a big entrée when we went out to dinner. When I wanted something with more substance, I ordered fish. I started eating only healthy whole grain cereals with fruit for breakfast. I stopped hitting fast-food drive-thrus when I was out running errands. Whenever I needed a quick meal out, I'd grab a sandwich. It wasn't easy to make these lifestyle changes, but I owe it to my kids."

And you owe it to yours. While you're cutting fat and cholesterol, try to also cut back on sugar. What Dr. Bob did may be impossible for most guys:

"I don't know how I did it; I just did. Six months ago, I stopped eating junk foods completely. Well, maybe 99 percent completely. No more cookies, ice cream, candy (my kids' Halloween stash is safe now), or chocolate. I even stopped putting sugar in my coffee. Now just so I don't go crazy I allow myself one vice: I'll eat any dessert my wife makes. This gives me a fix every couple of weeks or so."

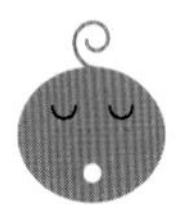

Making smart choices in the way you eat doesn't benefit only you. Your child is going to spend the next 18 years eating what you eat and learning good or bad eating habits from you. Teaching your child about good nutrition, and modeling it for her, will be a priceless gift she'll grow up to appreciate.

We're not suggesting that you go so far as to cut out almost all sweets. This isn't easy. But check your own intake of sugary foods, and make some changes if you feel inspired.

Another important thing we do is to pack our lunch for work each morning. If you wait until lunchtime to think about what to eat, you'll probably end up having fast food. Have a fast-food lunch every day, and you won't perform anywhere near your best, physically or mentally. It takes just a little planning to make a few days' worth of tuna salad or whatever your favorite healthy lunch food might be. You could also buy some frozen but relatively wholesome entrées from a health-food store. Skipping the fast food as much as possible makes all the difference in the world.

A few summers ago, a good friend of Dr. Jim's decided to get into better shape with a low-carb diet:

"I figured, 'Hey, if he can do it, I can do it better!' So, for several months, we were locked in a fierce battle of nerve, motivation, and self-control. We were sparring partners in the fight for our health. This was the first time in dozens of attempts that I actually started to lose weight. I couldn't believe it."

(Of course, low-carb diets may help you lose weight, but they shouldn't be an excuse for a high-fat diet of meat and cheese.)

Making smart choices in the way you eat doesn't benefit only you. Your child is going to spend the next 18 years eating what you eat and learning good or bad eating habits from you. Teaching your child about good nutrition, and modeling it for her, will be a priceless gift she'll grow up to appreciate (after she spends years whining because you won't feed her junk).

Something our dad passed on to us is his famous breakfast smoothie. It consists of milk, yogurt, tofu (you can't even taste it), honey, peanut butter (the natural kind), frozen bananas, blueberries, strawberries, and mango. That doesn't sound so bad, does it? But wait, there's more: oat bran, flax seed meal, soy protein powder, and a multi-nutrient smoothie powder mix. On most mornings we drink this breakfast on the way to work instead of coffee. This saves time and gives us a healthy energy boost. Even better is that our kids drink it, too (well, some of them). We thought Dad's smoothie was gross at first, but now we think it tastes great.

Another way you can take better care of yourself is to develop an exercise routine. This is just as important as eating well. You have to develop a plan that fits your interests: Are you competitive or not? Are you a morning person, or does your energy peak come later in the day? Our respective routines vary greatly, but we both manage to work out almost daily.

Dr. Bob isn't interested in working out at a health club:

"When I'm done with work, the last thing I want to do is go to a gym. But I decided to make better use of my free time in the early morning or at night, after the kids are in bed. I tried a treadmill, but it was too loud and a little rough on the feet. Then I bought an elliptical exercise machine. It's a cross between an exercise bike, a stair-climber, and a treadmill. You walk-run on

it, keeping your feet on the foot pads and pumping your arms back and forth. The best things about this machine are that it is quiet and that it fits right next to the couch in the living room. I started spending a half hour on the machine while watching TV every night. This worked perfectly for me. Now I do it every other morning before anyone else is up. It gives me a real boost of energy to start the day."

Exercise that gets your heart pumping but doesn't leave you exhausted is called cardiac aerobic exercise. You get your heart rate up to a certain level (which depends on your age) for a half hour, but you don't really tire yourself out too much. A half hour of such exercise four days a week is all you need to avoid that heart attack at age 55.

How does Dr. Jim say no to that double cheeseburger?

"I used to always say that I'd start eating right next year. But then I found an immediate motivation. About a year ago, I dusted off my old mountain bike and started riding again. With a sport like this, what you eat today affects how you perform—today! I never feel better than when I'm passing several other riders while going up a hill and not getting passed by anyone. Since I am very competitive by nature, I used this trait to my advantage in an area of my life in which I was failing miserably—my health. I try to get out on my bike for at least an hour on weekdays and for longer rides on weekends. Although my wife objects to my taking a half day off for golf or sailing, she understands that the

riding isn't just for fun. It's for our future."

Biking, like running, can be addictive—and that is great. The point is, you must do whatever it takes to motivate yourself to exercise. Having fun while doing it is an added bonus.

Think of healthy lifestyle changes you can make as a family. Take a family walk each week to the farmers' market to stock up on healthy produce. Shop at a health-food store instead of the regular grocery store. Find outdoor activities you both enjoy and can do with a baby (hiking, biking, jogging, swimming).

You know how people joked to your mate that she was "eating for two" when she was pregnant? Well, you are eating, and exercising, for three: yourself, your mate, and your baby. Your eating habits and lifestyle affect your entire family. Make some smart choices now while you are young. Start an exercise routine. If you need a little jump start, go get your cholesterol checked. We hope it isn't as high as Dr. Bob's was. If it is, better find out now while you're young enough to do something about it.

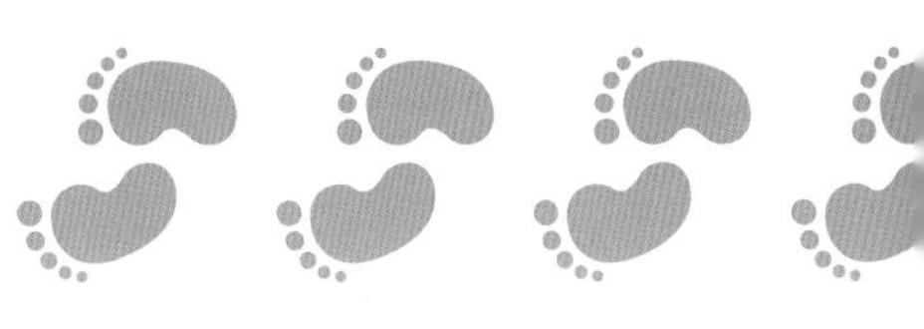

A Glimpse into the Future

The 25 tips you've just read are focused on helping a new father with his new family. But what about beyond the newborn time? We want to briefly discuss how early father-child bonding can evolve into a fulfilling long-term relationship.

Dr. Jim loves the movie *Father of the Bride* (the new version, with Steve Martin):

"For me, the best part of the movie is the relationship that the dad has with his twenty-something daughter. They shoot baskets and talk about their lives. She gives him big, warm hugs and still calls him Daddy. The movie doesn't show much about how this bond was formed. We doubt it started when the girl got to Little League age, when many men start to really get involved with their kids (if they aren't totally consumed by a career). More likely, such a close father-daughter relationship began very early, before she was old enough to remember."

A father is the most important man a child will ever know. Your son will spend much of his life striving to be just like you. Your daughter will likely seek a husband who reminds her of you. Who you are and how you behave will define, in your child's mind, the ideal man. This is a monumental responsibility, and you won't always be able to fulfill it. Sometimes you might yell when you should listen. You'll give in when you should stand firm. And once in a while you'll do something so idiotic that you'll feel like a complete failure as a father. Fortunately, you'll still be a superdad if you keep in mind some simple rules:

Give the gift of time. Set aside at least 15 minutes every day to read or play with your child. Offer a piggyback ride around the house, have a wrestling match on the living-room floor, or say a prayer together at bedtime. As your child gets older, you might sip hot chocolate together or share a hobby. Spending time with your child shows her that she is important to you.

Say "I love you" every day. Start this habit early in your child's life, and you will still be able to say "I love you" to your teenager without feeling awkward. Be generous with hugs and kisses. Even an occasional hand on the shoulder helps keep the two of you connected.

Try not to lose your temper with your child. Getting angry makes a child feel small and you even smaller. Count to 10 before you react. You want your child to respect you, not fear you.

Be generous with praise. Look for opportunities to give your child a pat on the back. Stick your child's drawings and report cards on the refrigerator. Don't miss those dance recitals or school plays.

Don't focus too much on winning. You don't want your child to think you pay attention or care only when she does well. Let her know that you enjoyed watching her even if her team lost, because she seemed to be having fun. Let her know that you love her for who she is, not just for what she can accomplish.

Well, that's it. We hope you've gained some insight into how to be the best dad you can be. We've tried to make it fun and humorous to keep you awake (there was humor in there, in case you missed it). We've attempted to approach fatherhood from every angle, including sports, sex, electronics, hobbies, exercise, careers, sex, money, food, playtime, housework (sorry), mothers-in-law (really sorry), tools, television, and sex (Oops! Cars, we forgot cars!). We trust that you, your mate, and your baby will be better off because of the time you've spent with us.

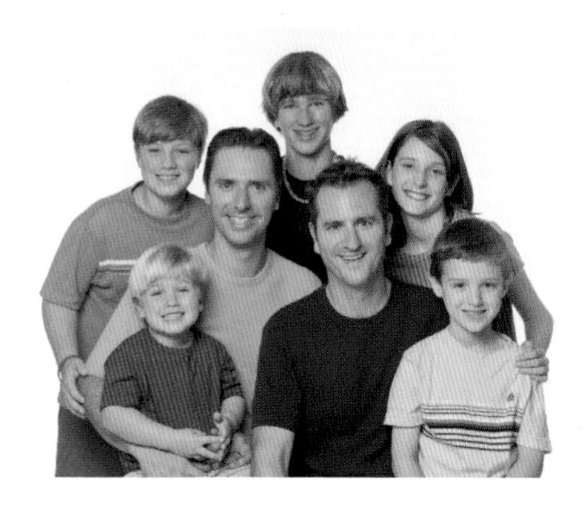

About the Authors

Robert W. Sears, M.D., and **James M. Sears, M.D.,** are pediatricians, authors, and fathers, and are the sons of venerable parenting experts and best-selling authors William and Martha Sears. They share a private pediatric practice with their father, are co-authors of *The Baby Book, The Premature Baby Book,* and *The Baby Sleep Book,* and have contributed to *Parenting* and *Baby Talk* magazines. Robert "Dr. Bob" lives with his wife and three children in Dana Point, California, and James "Dr. Jim" was co-host of the Emmy-winning *The Doctors* hit television show and lives with his family in Dana Point as well. Find the Sears Doctors online at www.AskDrSears.com. Their comprehensive website encompasses all aspects of parenting and pediatric medical care and offers family health news updates, seasonal medical alerts, personal stories about the doctors' lives in and out of the office, and answers to frequently asked questions.